Dolores Krieger, Ph.D., R.N., a professor of nursing at New York University, is noted for her study and development of therapeutic touch and has been explaining her healing techniques on radio and television throughout the country, in workshops, and in many published articles.

To Dora—from whom I have learned

DOLORES KRIEGER, PH.D., R.N.

The Therapeutic Touch

How to Use Your Hands to Help or to Heal

A FIRESIDE BOOK
Published by Simon & Schuster
New York London Toronto Sydney Tokyo Singapore

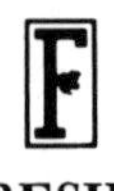

FIRESIDE
Simon & Schuster Building
Rockefeller Center
1230 Avenue of the Americas
New York, New York 10020

Published in 1986 by Prentice Hall Press
Originally published by Prentice-Hall, Inc.
First Fireside Edition 1992
Interior design by Claudia Citarella
Cover design by Tony Ferrara
Cover illustration by Mona Mark
Photographs by Janet Macrae
Illustrations (chapter 1) by Nabeela George

Manufactured in the United States of America

27 26 25

Library of Congress Cataloging-in-Publication Data

Krieger, Dolores.
The therapeutic touch.

Bibliography: p.
Includes index.
1. Mental healing. 2. Vital force—Therapeutic use. I. Title.
RZ401.K75 1979 615.8′51 79-4679
ISBN 0-671-76537-X

Contents

Preface

THERAPEUTIC TOUCH: HOW TO USE YOUR HANDS TO HELP OR TO HEAL has developed out of nine years of research on healing, six years of clinical practice of Therapeutic Touch, and five years of teaching, in modern dress, this very ancient practice. Four of these years of teaching have included a class at New York University, *Frontiers in Nursing: The Actualization of Potential for Therapeutic Human Field Interaction,* which was the first class of its kind in the United States squarely within a fully accredited curriculum for the master's degree. As of this date, almost 350 professional nurses have taken *Frontiers in Nursing* as part of their curriculum for either the M.A. or the Ph.D. degree, and I have taught another 4,000 professionals in the health field in continuing education programs at other universities in the United States and Canada and also

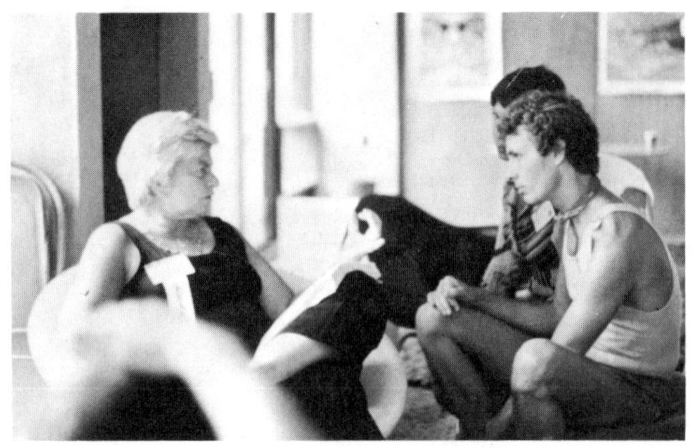

for professional organizations. Although I have taught comparatively few lay people, I recognized early that one need not be a professional person to be effective in the practice of Therapeutic Touch. I am thoroughly convinced that the ability to use Therapeutic Touch is a natural potential in man which can be actualized under the appropriate conditions, a now known fact to which the many uses it has been put to in both health facilities and homes over the past five years attest.

The sensitivity with which Therapeutic Touch responds to the human condition as a tool for healing rests firmly on the unique insights of Dora Kunz, who derived the techniques of Therapeutic Touch from the practice of the laying-on of hands; and I am deeply indebted to her for teaching me the most significant things I have learned about the healing process. This learning has matured through teaching others, and so for this opportunity I acknowledge my appreciation to "Krieger's Krazies," as the students who have taken the *Frontiers* course call themselves, and to "Krieger's Groupies," who have followed Therapeutic Touch workshop scheduling by plane, boat, and car. I have also been very fortunate to enjoy the support of and colleagial exchange with faculty at New York University and at other universities and with persons both in my own profession, nursing, and in other professions within the health field, for which I am happy to note my appreciation.

DOLORES KRIEGER, Ph.D., R.N.

1

Introduction

There are moments powerfully laden with thought which compress time a hundredfold. Such compression can happen with a glimpse of a most inconsequential gesture, as it did to me one midsummer morning quite recently. The gesture caught my eye as I leaned against a tree while surveying seven former students, each of whom was teaching a small cluster of workshop participants how to do Therapeutic Touch, a method (derived from the laying-on of hands) of using the hands to direct human energies to help or heal someone who is ill. At that particular moment each of the teachers was using her hands in an attempt to translate to her group something of the interior experience one has when playing the role of healer. As I scanned the seven group teachers, these gestures froze in my mind as a progression of living statues, and for a moment I felt a sense of déjà vu.

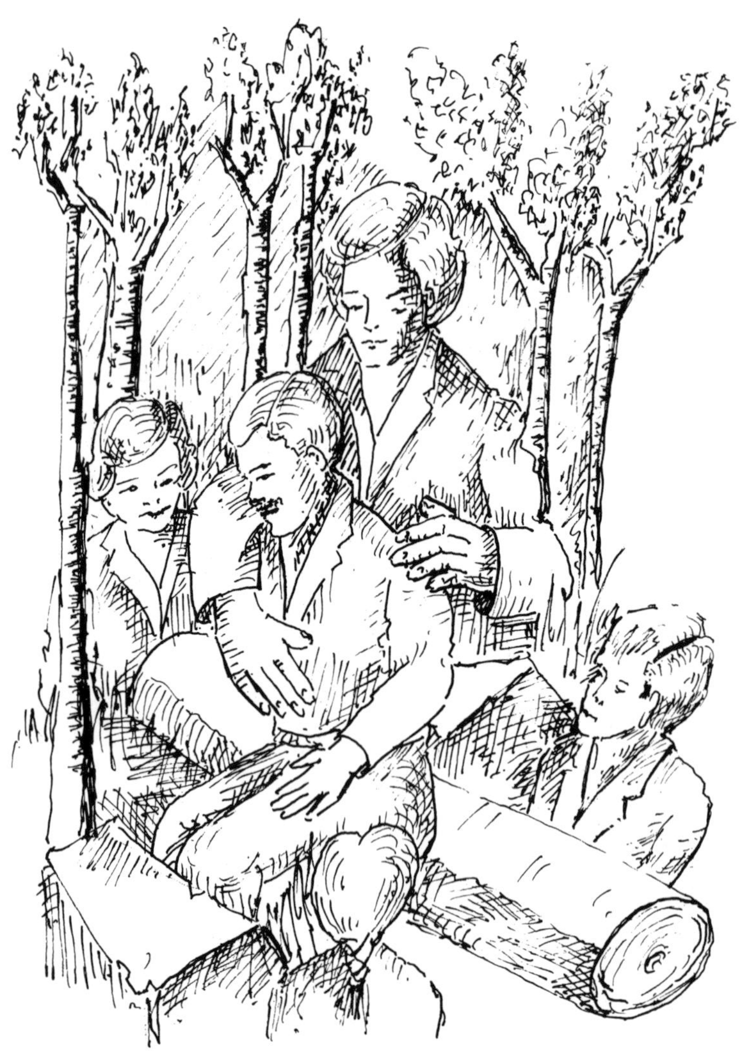

Each gesture was intimately known to me; each gesture called to mind an aspect of the working out from within of the highly personalized human interaction that is the healing act.

By turning my head slightly, I could see Mary and her group sitting on a log pile at the campfire site in the maple grove where we all were. She was teaching them how to center, how to reach deeply within, become aware of the facets of one's self, and then effortlessly bring those facets into alignment with each other. Deeper within the woods, Eloise was also teaching her group to center. She was talking about the importance of knowing and recognizing one's self in order to avoid the pitfall of mistaking all one's own problems for those of the healee's (patient's), or vice versa. In a clearing in the grove, Nancy was discussing the need to learn to put self aside and to give priority to meeting the needs of the healee. On the other side of the campfire site, Marianne was demonstrating to her group how to assess a person's field by becoming aware of energy differences without contacting the body with the hands. Sally was sitting against a tall silver maple tree; she was describing how she allows associative ideas to well up within her during the process of assessment. Farther in the woods, Janet was demonstrating Therapeutic Touch on a student who was sitting on a makeshift chair of logs. She was showing her group how to "unruffle" a person's field, or the area just beyond his skin, and how to clear seeming areas of congestion in this field until one feels a movement or flow of energy. Anna Marie, sitting with her group on the forest floor, was teaching them how to build up a localized field between the hands and then use it to transfer energy to the healee.

It happened that all of the teachers that day were nurses; however, I thought of the many hundreds—actually, almost four thousand at this writing—of students I have taught at universities and professional organizations around the country during the last five years. Although the majority of them were nurses, since touch is intrinsic in almost all phases of nursing practice, well over a thousand of those I had taught came from other professions or were laymen. Over the years, I have realized that only about four-fifths of those I've taught have gone on to incorporate Therapeutic Touch into their health care practices and that the other one-fifth treat the information as an intellectual exercise. However, of the larger percentage, I've only known of four persons who, when properly taught, were unable to do Therapeutic Touch. It does indeed seem to be a natural potential that can be actualized under the appropriate circumstances; and so as I looked at the students in the groups below me listening intently to their teachers, I realized that, if they were willing to give themselves adequate opportunities for practice, they would have this unique method of man caring for man literally at their fingertips in a short while.

Later on in the afternoon, my dog and I followed the headwaters of a nearby river to the cool shade of a gorge overhung with ancient hemlocks and large beech trees. As I recalled the morning's events with the intention of picking up anything that might need elaboration in that evening's workshop discussion, I thought again of the students and reminisced over the days of my own beginning knowledge about the therapeutic use of hands.

My interest in the therapeutic use of hands came originally through research and, very importantly, from a lady, Dora Kunz, who has been a very significant person in my life. Dora, as she is affectionately known, was born with a unique ability to perceive subtle energies around living beings. From the time she was a child, she studied the function and control of these energies under the tutelage of Charles W. Leadbeater, one of the great seers of the twentieth century. Through the years, she has studied these abilities in depth so that they have become like a fine instrument in her hands which she can turn on or off at will. During this time, she has worked closely with many medical doctors and scientists, sharing with them her special point of view. When I first met her, she was studying the processes involved in the healing act with several of them.[1] They were studying many healers, among them Oskar Estebany, a world renowned healer.[2]

Oskar Estebany had been a Colonel in the Hungarian cavalry. He loved horses; and one day, when his own horse became ill, he stayed all night in the stable with the horse. He knew the horse would be shot if it did not recover, and so he did everything he could think of to help the horse: He massaged it, he caressed it, he talked to it, he prayed over it. The last, in particular, he did not do lightly, for he was a man of deep religious beliefs. In the morning, to the surprise of all, including himself, Estebany found that the horse was well.

After that incident, when other horses became ill, the cavalrymen would bring their horses to Estebany and he would help them as he could. In time, the children of the cavalrymen would bring their sick pets to Estebany to be healed, and he became very well known for this ability.

Mr. Estebany thought he could heal only animals, he once told me, until one Sunday morning when a child in a neighbor's house became very ill. The family was unable to contact a doctor for some reason; and finally, in desparation, the father grabbed up the child and ran with him to Estebany's house to ask him to do to his child what he was able to do to horses. At first, Estebany refused because he did not think his method of healing would work on humans; but the father persisted in his request, and finally Estebany treated the child. The child got better, and Estebany continued to work with people until he retired from the cavalry. Upon his

[1] Shafika Karagulla, *Breakthrough to Creativity* (Los Angeles: De Vorss and Co., 1967), pp. 123–146.

[2] D.M. Rorvik, "The Healing Hand of Mr. E.," *Esquire* 81 February 1974.: 70, 154, 156, 159–160.

retirement, he decided to offer his services for research purposes; and so, after a chain of events that saw him leave Hungary and take up residence in Canada, he joined the group with whom Dora was studying the process of the healing act.

At the completion of that study, Dora, Estebany, and a medical doctor, Otelia Bengssten, M.D., decided to do a further study on a large sample of medically referred patients. Since I am a nurse, and since I had just received my Ph.D. degree, I was asked to join them. The study took place in the foothills of the Berkshires where the facilities could handle not only all of us but also the patients in residence.

My duties were actually peripheral to the study per se; and in retrospect, I realize that this was a good thing, for it gave me both an opportunity to observe Estebany close-up and the time in which to observe him. It is almost funny to recall that what I saw was not much of what I had anticipated—incantations, the waving of arms, and a hypnotic glare in the eye of the healer was what my occasional readings had prepared me for. Instead, I found that Estebany was a well-built man with cheery blue eyes and a frequent smile. His healing ability carried with it a deep sense of commitment, and he did not spare himself in its practice: He frequently worked on the healees sixteen hours a day; more often than not he worked until Dora took away his patients and made him relax. Even then, he would take with him rolls of cotton batting to "magnetize" for the healees, and in the morning he would be up before sunrise, ready to start healing again. He would distribute the magnetized cotton to the healees after having it near his person during the night; some of these patients have told me that, even after nearly a year, they could still feel an energy flow from the cotton.

During the healing sessions, Estebany was very quiet; he would sit next to the healee and do exactly what he purported to do—lay his hands on the patient. Although he made every effort to put the healee at ease, there was little conversation, for his command of the English language was limited, even though he spoke several other languages fluently. He would most frequently sit on a small stool either in front of or behind the healee and put his hands wherever he felt they were needed; occasionally Dora would suggest that he put his hands over a particular area that she could perceive in need of being energized. At times, he would make a little joke to put the healee at ease, but other than that he would remain with his hands on the healee, occasionally shifting position or placing his hands on another area, the entire treatment lasting for about twenty to twenty-five minutes. The healee would then leave the room, to come back the next day if his or her condition warranted it.

Estebany's actions seemed so simple that I began interactional sketches and behavioral profiles of both the healer and the healees, thinking that I would capture some of the subtleties I felt must be going on. As I carefully tried to record the physical activities the healer engaged in and the nonverbal as well as the verbal behavior of both healer and healee, it soon became apparent to me that the postures were but gross outer expressions of what appeared to be an intense interior experience for both of them. When pressed, Estebany would say that he felt that he was a channel for the spirit of Jesus the Christ; and when questioned, his patients would say that they felt heat from Estebany's hands and that they felt relaxed. The healees did indeed seem relaxed, and there was a noticeable up-welling of vibrant energy that seemed to come from his person as the days went by; and, in addition, a felt energetic intensity built up in the rooms in which he did his healing, so that it was quite perceptible upon entering the house.

I was impressed with Dora's descriptions of her perceptions of the healees' pathology descriptions, which might well have been taken out of Spalteholz-Spanner's *Atlas of Human Anatomy* or Guyton's *Textbook of Medical Physiology,* both classics in their field and neither of which she had ever read. It was as though she were perceiving directly the inner functions and dysfunctions of the patient. In actuality, she went further than either Spalteholz-Spanner or Guyton in her perceptions; but more often than chance could account for, her logic was irrefutable, and the consequent history of the patient bore her judgments out. On the other hand, if she didn't know or wasn't sure, she would say so, flat out. It was this precision that made her so invaluable to the scientists and doctors she worked with, and I myself learned a great deal from her wisdom.

Over the course of the study, some of the patients reported that they felt better; but there were no miraculous cures except one that could be termed "instantaneous," and that cure occurred in a seemingly mundane fashion. One of the participants in the healing sessions was a well-groomed attractive lady in early middle age. She was a nice lady, but there was little about her that one would recognize as being unusual. I believe that she came because a friend was coming to the sessions; and she did the kinds of things the other people did upon coming out to that part of the country—walk down to see the falls, chat, play bridge, plan to go antiquing. For several years, she had had a boutique on a luxury liner that plied the Caribbean Sea. One day, during a heavy storm, she was thrown against a bulkhead and sustained injuries to her head. She was left with an inner ear syndrome that seriously interfered with her sense of balance. In the intervening years, she had had exhaustive work-ups from fifteen medical personnel, including six medical specialists who now felt there was nothing more that could be done; and so she had come with her friend to see Estebany.

Her first treatment was late in the afternoon, and I remember her coming into the house somewhat hesitantly. She was soon made at ease, and Estebany treated her for about twenty-five minutes. After her treatment, she sat on the lawn and chatted, had dinner, and went to bed somewhat earlier than usual. In the morning, she came down to breakfast and said quietly, "I think I feel better." The medical doctor reexamined her and had her try to precipitate the feelings she had previously had, but to no avail; she was indeed cured and has remained so over the past nine intervening years.

For the rest of the healees, this was not the case; however, in the weeks to come I was to be astounded by the number of medical reports or first person reports that told either of an amelioration of symptoms or of an actual disappearance of symptoms. Part of my surprise was based on the complicated nature of the medical diagnoses of the healees in the sample. These diagnoses covered all known systems of the body: Pancreatitis, brain tumor, emphysema, multiple endocrine disorders, rheumatoid arthritis, and congestive heart disease were but a few. There was nothing in either my previous education or experience by which I could rationalize these results. I went back to my behavioral profiles and interactional sketches and reexamined them. After considerable analysis, I realized that the only thing that importantly intervened between Estebany and the healees was touch by the laying-on of his hands, and I decided to do postdoctoral research on this healing process.

The discussion of my subsequent studies and those of others I will leave to a later chapter. At this time, I will only mention that I found that when ill people are treated by the laying-on of hands, a significant change occurs in the hemoglobin component of their red blood cells. The healing sessions continued over several summers with Estebany, and during this time he was the healer in my pilot study and in two of the subsequent large-scale studies I did. The point I want to make here is that, as I learned to tighten the control of my studies, my appreciation for the validity of healing by the laying-on of hands also increased, and I became interested in learning whether I could do it too.

Estebany did not feel that people could be taught how to heal; rather, he felt that they had to be born with the gift, and he never responded to persons' requests that he teach them. Dora thought differently and, therefore, began a workshop which she opened to all who wished to learn how to heal, and I was one of those students.

Dora was a tough but very good teacher. She was not afraid of experimenting. She would have two or three of us work together while she would perceive how the interaction went. If we ourselves did not understand what it was we were doing or the effect we were having on our healees, we were free to question her as we went along. Dora would describe her perceptions to the best of her ability and the limits of our understanding. This last was most important, for, although we engage in interrelationships with others constantly, we are not always aware of our unconscious involvements and motivation–of the projections of our shadow that lurk behind the mask of the persona–nor are we aware of the potent effect these behaviors have on others. Dora's point of view always stemmed from an utterly honest ethical base, and so she made us look at these hidden aspects of ourselves and recognize their involvement in our motivations to play the role of healer. On the other hand, she was never adamant that we do things one way or another; she always emphasized that she was experimenting in this kind of healing too, and that we had to make individual decisions for and about ourselves. Dora also helped us sensitize ourselves to our human frailities and limitations. For instance, at one point when we were experimenting on the use of mantras (sounds which convey specific vibrational effects), we all felt uncomfortable at the sounds of our first expressions, which were by no means melodious. Immediately after our first attempts, Dora's comment put us at ease so that we could bear these initial efforts with impersonal equanimity: "Of course," she quietly said, "Psychologically, you first have to get used to making the sound–that there is a unison in the emotions as well as in the sound itself. . . . I think it is nice to do it all together; after all, it's the opportunity for coming together in an emotional unity that is important."

Similarly, we experimented with the use of the hands in the transfer of human energies. I think that in this case also it was through the model of Dora patiently accepting us as we were that we learned to tolerate, then to accept, and finally to help each other in our first clumsy attempts at healing. We found that our combined efforts could be synergistic in helping people who were ill, and so frequently two or more of us would work simultaneously as a team on the same patient. In learning to link up with each other in this mutual undertaking, we found that we also exercised our innate sense of timing, both in reference to each other and in reference to the healee. I have since come to appreciate the centrality of this increased acuity in timing during the healing act, for the sense of timing is crucial throughout the process and is, I think, a major factor in making the process of healing an holistic act.

Dora fostered these group activities, and she usually directed her remarks to us as a group, rather than individually, except at our own request. One morning toward the middle of the first workshop, she happened to be telling us that we were not doing something correctly. At that time, we were blindfolding the healees so that they could not tell who was working on them. One of the healees suddenly spoke out and said, "No, Dora, that isn't entirely so. I always know when Dee (myself) is working on me. I can tell exactly where her hands are from the deep heat that is generated inside my body, and I can feel the energy flow she transmits to me." I was amazed by what Helga said and realized that I was so intent on what I was trying to do that I had no idea of whether what she said was so or not. The subject turned to something else, and we went on; however, Helga came up to me later and described more explicitly what she had experienced when I was working on her. This feedback was most helpful for me to understand the experience in which I was involved in the healing act.

I began to draw on this understanding by trying to sensitize myself to any changes occurring in the healees I worked with and by listening carefully to any verbal feedback they offered me. I also availed myself of every opportunity that presented itself to exercise the therapeutic use of hands, and I began to gain a repertoire of experiences from which I could draw a deeper understanding of the healing act per se.

In retrospect, I see that I was very lucky to be engaged in both research and teaching at the same time that I was learning clinical applications of the therapeutic use of hands, for the research and teaching fostered an objectivity that stood me in very good stead during the practice of this highly personalized human interaction. I developed a method of looking over my own shoulder, so to speak, so that I could consciously understand the subtle dynamics of my practice; and this was very useful a few years later when I developed a curriculum for the first course on the therapeutic use of hands to be squarely included within a university master's level program in this country.

I had a second opportunity for reliable feedback about nine months later when Dora and I were invited to a conference in Council Grove, Kansas that was cosponsored by the Menninger Foundation and the Association for Transpersonal Psychology. It happened that about eight or nine of us were into healing of one kind or another, and so Elmer Green, Ph.D., Director of Research at Menninger's and the prime mover in the Council Grove Conferences, asked us if we would be willing to take part in a small study. Dora, Jack Schwarz, who is a well-known psychic, and I volunteered, and a core of five medical doctors made up a panel to evaluate us.

By prearrangement, a patient was brought in from a hospital in Topeka, together with his physician. Each of the three of us was assigned a person to act as scribe and given fifteen minutes to be alone with the patient. The protocol allowed us to do anything we wished to the patient except talk to him. Both while in the room and afterward, we dictated our impressions about the history and condition of the patient to our individual scribes. In the meantime, the panel of medical doctors met with the patient's physician and reviewed the patient's medical records. When we were finished, the panel then took our scribes' reports; matched them against the medical findings, laboratory reports, and so on; and evaluated each of us. Dora and Jack were correct in their impressions, and each received a 100% rating. I received 80% as my rating, which was considerably beyond my expectations. I learned a great deal from this experience, and it served to bolster my self-confidence considerably.

As my interest in healing deepened, I began to realize that healing offered a rich source for the study of man. I found myself challenged by the question: Why is touch therapeutic?—a question which has stimulated a continuing quest. I had always read omnivorously, and I now redoubled my efforts, but with discretion. My research and the healing act itself served to channel the direction of my search, but this search nonetheless covered a very broad scope. Happily, Fritz L. Kunz, Dora's husband, was one of the first persons in education to recognize the need for an integration of concepts in this day of mounting floods of facts; and over the years I learned from him how to draw relationships between isolated facts as I read and so to integrate large bodies of information. I had had a very good background in the life sciences, particularly in neurophysiology, which I

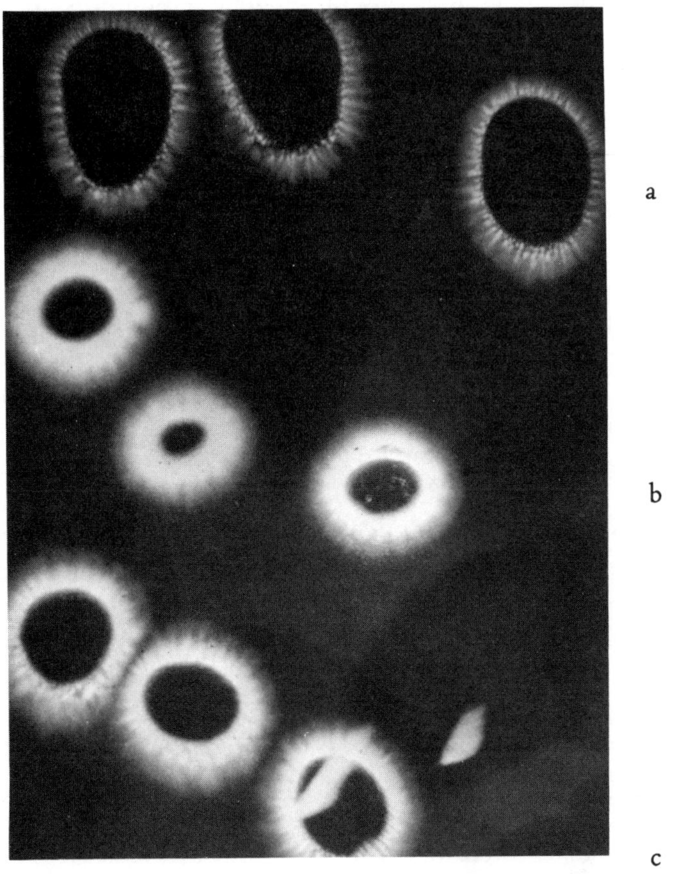

a

b

c

Live Kirlian photography (a television first). The three middle fingers: (a) normal state; (b) during therapy; and (c) after therapy.

had taught for several years, and this was very helpful as I began to look into the health practices of yoga and at the readings in Aruvedic medicine, Tibetan medicine, and, more recently, Chinese medicine. The alternate views these bodies of literature held from those I had learned in my formal education became understandable on my own terms only as I gave myself to in depth explorations of the nuances and overtones with which the apparent meanings of terms or phrases used in these cultures were clothed. One such instance is the subsystem of energy which is called *prana* in Sanskrit, which my research had led me to believe to be at the base of the human energy transfer in the healing act. It does not have an adequate translation in English, primarily because our culture does not understand energy within the same context as does the Eastern world. Most often, *prana* is translated as vigor or vitality; however, an analysis of the literature indicates that the term really pertains to the organizing factors that underlie what we call the life process. *Prana*, therefore, is responsible for such phenomena as regeneration and wound healing. Further, one begins to find out that *prana* is related to the element *Vayu* (Sanskrit), which is concerned with air but, more importantly, also with motion. It is thus that one begins to see that *prana* is not related to the respiratory act in a simple breathing-in and breathing-out fashion, but that it is a principle underlying the rhythmic movement that makes breathing imperative, whether it is the breathing that occurs in the lungs or the chemical reciprocity that goes on at a molecular level in the rhythmical interchange of oxygen and carbon dioxide during the respiratory process at the cellular level while the organism is alive.

As one goes deeper into the study of *prana,* one finds that the literature of these ancient people makes statements that can be in consonance with some of the most contemporary theory of the West. The literature of the East, for instance, says that *prana* derives from the sun. This statement is not at all at variance with our current recognition that the crucial chemical base of the life process in man is dependent upon sunlight, for the photons coming from the sun set off the process of photosynthesis, which is the driving force for the primary synthesis of organic matter. When one considers that the process begins with inorganic matter, the statement sounds more like a miracle than do the ancient texts of the East!

The Eastern literature also says that normally healthy people have an excess of *prana.* Again, I find their statement acceptable, for the best of our Western texts on physiology tells us that there is a great deal of redundancy in the human body. If the body is damaged in any way—let us take the instance of a heart attack—many compensatory body mechanisms come into play: Within thirty seconds autonomic circulatory reflexes begin to compensate for the failure of the heart muscle to function properly; concomitantly, the body chemistry begins an holistic adjustment of fluids and electrolytes directed by the adrenals as well as other endocrine glands, and structural changes occur in the blood components, stimulating and being stimulated by principles of repatterning as a new collateral blood supply starts to position itself into the space of the damaged tissues (another "miracle" for which we in the West do not give ourselves credit).[3] To go a bit further: In the East they say that persons who are ill have a deficit of this energy, *prana;* and the lassitude that accompanies illness would seem to give evidence to support this. Another statement, that *prana* can be transferred from one individual to another, may not be so readily apparent to us unless we have gotten into the practice and literature of hatha yoga, tantric yoga, or the martial arts of the Orient. We can, however, in these days of potent theatrical and television personalities, recognize this phenomenon as charisma and give it credence in that guise. If one is willing to go so far and, in addition, is willing to accept one basic assumption—that man is an open system—then it is not difficult to consider the following model seriously: Conceive of the healer as an individual whose health gives him access to an overabundance of *prana* and whose strong sense of commitment and intention to help ill people gives him or her a certain control over the projection of this vital energy. The act of healing, then, would entail the channeling of this energy flow by the healer for the well-being of the sick individual. If we posit an open system, then we recognize that the healer, like every man, is in constant energetic flux—that is, energetically, he is in a constant state of energy in-put, through-put, and out-put. All of this is actually a continued constant flow, a process, rather than separate states: He/she is what Sherrington called ". . .but an eddy in a constant stream."[4] Following a logical deduction from this model, one can also recognize that, although the healer projects this energy, *prana,* for the use of another person, the healer himself is not depleted or deprived of energy unless he identifies himself too closely with the process. This last has complex psychodynamic implications that we shall explore more fully later in this book, but it is well to look at this rationale now. Where one stands in relation to the personal question, Why do I want to play the role of healer? is crucial to what one does with the process of healing and—importantly—to what the process of healing does to the individual so engaged.

As I sat with my dog, Jocko, that day at the bottom of the gorge and recalled the incidents I've related above, I watched the river swirling about the rocks in midstream. Thoughts of Sherrington's analogy to man as but an "eddy" came to mind, and once again I wondered—I still wonder—Why do I want to play the role of healer? Like the river's waters swirling

[3] Arthur C. Guyton, *Textbook of Medical Pharmacology* (Philadelphia: W.B. Saunders Co., 1961), pp. 301-18.

[4] C. Sherrington, *Man On His Nature* (Garden City, N.Y.: Doubleday, 1955), p. 83.

at my feet, I realized that this question had many levels of expression and, similarly, that its answers are equally multifaceted and probably dependent upon the psychological depth at which one can confront one's self. However, the act of importance is to be willing to begin the confrontation; and so I invite the reader to join me in this quest in the following pages as we look behind the "why" to the roots of the healing act, to what it seems to be, to how each of us may do it, and as we begin to explore together what it may do to and for each of us.

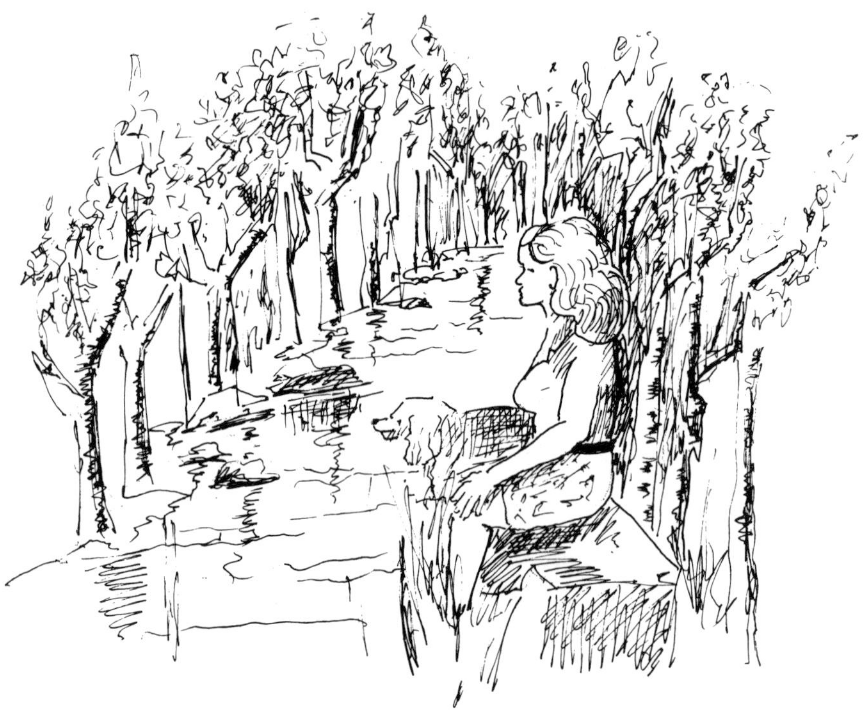

2

Healing as a Natural Potential

Can you heal? History gives evidence that you can.

The therapeutic use of hands is an exceedingly ancient example of man's ability to help man. There is a written history of it that goes back some 5,000 years, and there is pictoral evidence in cave paintings in the Pyrenees that have been estimated to date back 15,000 years. Evidence of its use is demonstrated in the ancient traditions which continue to be handed down from teacher to pupil in India, Tibet, and China; in the early rock carvings of Egypt and Chaldea; in the writings of both the old and the new Judeo-Christian testaments; and in the accounts of certain historical figures, such as the Roman emperors Vespasian and Hadrian, or the Norwegian King Olaf, who was thought by some to have been a saint. In fact, the laying-on of hands was known as the "King's Touch" in early

France and England; the touch of the kings of that period was considered especially good for the curing of goiter and other throat ailments. There are actual instances recorded where more common folk of that day who were also able to demonstrate this ability were suspected of being pretenders to the throne.

During the Middle Ages, innumerable accounts of healing by laying-on of hands appear in church histories in the West. It is, however, a sad commentary on these times to note that healing outside the church was looked upon with suspicion and thought to be witchcraft, imprecations of the devil, or, at best, mere nonsense. Translations of Cabeza de Vaca, who recorded the explorations of the Spanish conquistadors of the early sixteenth century, wrote about the native Americans in southwestern North America:

> On an island of which I have spoken, they wished to make us physicians without examination or inquiring for diplomas. They cure by blowing upon the sick, and with that breath and the imposing of hands they cast out infirmity. They ordered that we also should do this and be of use to them in some way. We laughed at what they did, telling them that it was folly, that we knew not how to heal. . . .[1]

The therapeutic use of hands, therefore, appears to be a universal human act; however, it is an act that we have all but forgotten in this scientific age in our adulation of things mechanical, synthetic, and, frequently, antihuman. Therapeutic Touch has recaptured this simple but elegant ancient mode of healing and mated it with the rigor and power of modern science; there is hard evidence that treatment by Therapeutic Touch affects the healee's (patient's) blood components[2] and brain waves,[3] and that it elicits a generalized relaxation response.[4] Interestingly,

[1] F.W. Hodge and T. Lewis, *Spanish Explorers in the Southwestern United States* (New York: Barnes and Noble, 1970), p. 52.

[2] Dolores Krieger, "The Relationship of Touch, with Intent to Help or Heal, to Subjects' In-vivo Hemoglobin Values: A Study in Personalized Interaction," (Paper delivered at the American Nurses Association Ninth Nursing Research Conference, San Antonio, Texas, March 21–23, 1973, American Nurses Association, 1974) pp. 39–58.

[3] Erik Peper and Sonia Ancoli, "The Two Endpoints of an EEG Continuum of Meditation" (Paper presented at Biofeedback Society of America Conference, Orlando, Florida, March 1977).

[4] Dolores Krieger, "Therapeutic Touch: A Mode of Primary Healing Based on a Holistic Concern for Man," *The Journal for Holistic Medicine* 1 (1975), pp. 6–10.

there are also strong indications that this highly personalized interaction invokes in the healee a sense of self-responsibility for his or her health. These various effects will be considered in later chapters, but the point I want to bring to your attention now is that since Therapeutic Touch derives from a mode of healing that persons of all cultures since the dawn of documented history have been able to use, *you,* too, can learn to heal.

This is not an idle statement. As you read this book, I think you will be impressed that there is little I have to teach you that you haven't done before at some time in your life. It is a misconception, for instance, to think that you have to work up a lather of complex activity to generate the energy that is transferred to the healee during the healing act. I am quite convinced that the major expertise of the healer is not centered in such efforts, but rather that the expertise lies in the healer's ability to *direct* energies, and that is what you must learn if you would play the role of healer.

Therapeutic Touch is noticeably useful for two things: It elicits a rather profound, generalized relaxation response in the healee, and it is very good at relieving pain. It may come as a surprise that healing is not mentioned, since that is ostensibly a major purpose of Therapeutic Touch. However, as you yourself will find out once you get into the practice of Therapeutic Touch, in almost every case there comes a moment when it must be acknowledged that it is the patient who heals himself. The transfer of energy from the person playing the role of healer is most usually little more than a booster until the patient's own recuperative system takes over. At best, the healer accelerates the healing process. You will find, however, that the range of circumstances under which Therapeutic Touch can be helpful is very large. To give you an idea of how Therapeutic Touch works, I will describe several cases which occurred to students like yourself during the past few months.

I am sure you can relate to Susan's experience. Susan and Robert had recently had their first baby, a boy. They had divided up the necessary chores so that Susan found that she was able to resume her classes at the university. One of the courses she took was taught by me and included information on Therapeutic Touch as one of the modes of human field interaction. Robert, a tough-minded engineer, was skeptical when Susan told him about the course, and he told her frankly that he thought she was wasting her money.

The baby grew and started to teethe. One night the baby woke up crying in pain. It happened to be Robert's turn to get up and try to soothe the child, and so he walked the baby, cuddled it, and sang to it.

But it was all to no avail: The baby let its feelings be known in a continued high-pitched wail.

Finally, Susan could stand it no longer. She got out of bed and took the child from Robert, saying, "Let me show you something I learned about Therapeutic Touch today." She moved her hands in a manner we've come to call "unruffling the field," in which it is thought that what feels like a congestion in the body energies can be swept out of a person's field with a motion away from the surface of the body. After this motion has been made several times, one frequently feels a normal energetic flow quite rapidly replace the static build-up. With the conclusion of the motion, the baby suddenly stopped crying, gave his mother a wide-eyed gaze as if amazed, laid his head on her shoulder, and immediately fell asleep. Robert, who was looking on intently, opened his mouth and closed it twice, shook his head, and sat down—hard. The next week, after leaving the child with a baby sitter, a radiant Susan turned up at class with Robert at her elbow.

Babies respond very well to Therapeutic Touch. As will be noted in a later chapter, one of the keys to the successful treatment of children is to do the healing act gently and for a very short period of time. We have had particular success in using Therapeutic Touch to support the growth and development of babies who are born prematurely. The following story is about a student in another class, one that has a very long title, but which I call Space-time Matrices of Human Development.

I teach this class on Thursday evening. At the end of the first class, a student came up to me and told me that she was pregnant. She said that her "due date" would occur during the time set aside for final examinations and asked whether arrangements could be made for her to take the exam prior to the winter recess. We made this arrangement and parted. The Thursday before the Thanksgiving holiday, the student intercepted me in the corridor after class. I hardly recognized her, for there were dark circles under her eyes, her hair was disheveled, and she was obviously emotionally distraught. As we rode down in the elevator, she told me that her baby had been born much too prematurely and that its birth weight was only two pounds, six ounces. She said, "Dr. Krieger, I was wondering if you would be willing to come to the hospital with me and put your hands on my baby?" I realized that she had more of a need to touch her baby than I, for at that weight there was a strong possibility that the child might die; if it lived, the probability of multiple congenital malformations was high, so that physiologically the baby's development would have a very stormy course. Either way, it was important for her to do all she could for her baby, and so I asked, "Wouldn't you like to learn to do Therapeutic Touch for your baby?" The look in her face was answer enough; and when the elevator reached the main floor, we both went in search of a quiet spot.

New York University is the largest private university in the United States, and it is not an easy place in which to find a quiet spot, particularly between class changes. However, we did manage to find a tiny alcove, and I taught her what I could of Therapeutic Touch in the short time we had together. When I was satisfied that she was able to do the techniques and to understand the dynamics of what she was doing, we parted.

The next week's class fell on the Thanksgiving holiday, and so we did not see each other for two weeks. As I entered the classroom on that evening, again, I hardly recognized her, for she was radiantly happy as she told me of her experience with Therapeutic Touch.

Her baby was in an Isolette, which is an enclosed criblike box that allows a controlled supply of oxygen and temperature. It also has two snugly fitting portholes through which one can put one's hands, and so she had no difficulty in doing Therapeutic Touch to her baby in a natural manner under the circumstances. What called her to the attention of the doctors and nurses in that "preemie" unit was her son's unexpected weight gain and concomitant neurological progress. The baby now weighed three pounds, eight ounces, and the doctors and nurses questioned her in surprise at the baby's accelerated behavioral profile. She, however, was not surprised. Cooly, she told them, "Of course. I've been doing Dr. Krieger's Therapeutic Touch to my baby." Of course "Dr. Krieger's Therapeutic Touch" meant nothing at all to them; and so they questioned her further, became intrigued, and finally asked her to teach it to them, which she did. By the end of the day, the whole "preemie" staff was doing Therapeutic Touch. Interestingly, in a day or so the parents of the other preemies raised a complaint: The babies, after all, belonged to them; surely they should be taught how to enhance their own babies' development. To meet this request, my student extended her teaching to the parents; and in a short time it was incorporated as general procedure on this preemie unit, a unit that is one of the largest of its kind in the world.

Some time later, at a class time that I give over to the students, she decided that she wanted to tell the story to the other students. By chance, one of these students was pregnant and gave birth the following February to a premature child. This mother now decided to do Therapeutic Touch on her baby, with consequences very similar to the experience related above—the only difference was that this mother gave birth to her child in a large private hospital, while the first mother gave birth in a large city hospital. Nevertheless, the second mother was again asked to teach the doctors and the nurses in that hospital's preemie unit; and, again, the mothers of the other babies in that unit asked to be taught Therapeutic Touch, and, again, Therapeutic Touch was incorporated into the unit's procedures.

The ability of Therapeutic Touch to alleviate pain rapidly is striking. Dora Kunz, the lady who taught me the most valuable things I know about healing, once remarked that if Therapeutic Touch did nothing more for terminally ill patients with cancer than alleviate their pain, it would be a worthwhile effort, and I thoroughly agree with her. The insidious effects of pain can be devastating to the personality faced with a medical diagnosis that offers little hope. The relief from pain does at least give one time to compose oneself for traversing a territory that is still little explored.

Another area that is in need of further exploration by the health sciences is that of psychogenic diseases. Prime among these may be asthma. Some time ago, I found that asthma is very responsive to Therapeutic Touch. Upon that occasion I was having acupuncture treatments for a complicated knee condition for which I have been unable to treat myself, and I came in for my first treatment to find the acupuncturist in the midst of a severe asthmatic attack. When my own treatment was over, he allowed me to do Therapeutic Touch to him. By chance, my wristwatch was clearly visible to me during the entirety of the treatment, and so I can accurately state the length of time it took for the asthmatic attack to cease: four minutes. The second time I visited this acupuncturist, some days later, he was in the throes of an extremely severe asthmatic attack: The dyspnea was considerably labored, the wheezes were pronounced, and his complexion was ashen. I again treated him, and within two and a half minutes his attack subsided. The rapidity with which Therapeutic Touch frequently works makes me believe that whatever time scale Therapeutic Touch operates in, it is not our linear tick-tock clock time.

The deeper one studies the dynamics of healing, the more one is impressed by how little we really know about the healing act. I would like to tell you of one other incident that will, I think, give some indication of another area of knowledge that still eludes us. This incident happened on the last day of an end-of-summer workshop series that I gave on the campus of the School of Medicine at the University of California at San Diego two years previous to this writing.

I was crossing the campus one morning on the way to my class when I heard my name called and turned to see that the caller was a well-dressed man in a wheelchair who was rapidly and expertly propelling the wheelchair over the campus grounds in my direction. I stepped through a small flower garden and met him. He told me that he had had a transected spinal cord and that he was paralyzed. Recently, the heel of his right foot had developed a decubital ulcer, something that most paralytic persons fear, since it can ground them in bed and cause serious physiological sequelae. He knew nothing of me; however, in one of the classes he was taking on campus my name and the course that I was teaching on healing was mentioned. He had tried to reach me several times, and now he felt desperate, since he knew that that day would be my last on campus.

A quick glance at my watch told me that I had very little time before class, and so I decided to try to help him right there. I bent down, put my books on the sidewalk, picked up his leg, and rested it on my own knee. As I did so, I felt the hard, unresisting metal of his long leg braces under his pants and saw the thick leather of his shoes that kept his helpless feet in postural alignment. To my surprise, however, I quickly felt the heat of his injured tissues; other signs also guided me to the troubled areas and indicated the progressive effect of Therapeutic Touch. In a minute or two, he began to describe the heat that he felt from the treatment, and he was able to tell me what part of the tissues he felt it in. His voice level was very low as he spoke to me; and, very shortly, he remarked how relaxed he felt. When I realized that I had done as much as I could for him at that time, I got up, and we bid each other farewell.

I hurried across the campus to my class; but as I did so, I was aware that something bothered me. Halfway to the class, I suddenly stopped in midpath, realizing what it was that had been struggling to rise to consciousness: That fellow had had no idea of what to expect from Therapeutic Touch, and yet he had described exactly the sensations other healed persons had reported as their reactions to Therapeutic Touch. The big difference—and this realization made me reach out to a nearby tree as its implications dawned on me—was that, unlike the many other people, this fellow's spinal cord was severed, and thus he did not have the neural circuits to relay the sensations he described to me. I have always had a special interest in neurology and, indeed, had taught neurophysiology and neuroanatomy at the graduate level. I found myself visualizing the damage indicated by that man's history as I analyzed the probable consequences of his damaged neural circuitry. Slowly, reluctantly, the left side of my brain admitted ignorance, and the right brain took advantage of the momentary break in attention to thrust an heuristic "ah-ha" at my consciousness. The nervous system you are thinking of, it said, is a three-dimensional net. What the data that you are analyzing so squarely means is that, however that young man sensed those feelings he described, his sensing was other than three-dimensional!

That, of course, was the case, and my experiences since than have confirmed it to my own inner satisfaction. It is a bit scary to think in these terms, but it is also exhilarating to foretaste the adventure that lies ahead in the continuing exploration of the healing act.

You can be part of this adventure. You can heal. My experience has convinced me that the potential to heal lies latent in persons who are willing to reach beyond themselves in their attempts to help others—that is, those who have a deep intentionality to heal, a strong motivation in the interest of meeting the needs of others (rather than just bolstering the needs of his or her own ego structure), and the ability to honestly confront the question, *Why* do I want to play the role of healer? If you have these characteristics, you can heal. In the following pages, I'd like to help you on your way.

3

The Laboratory of the Self

The functional basis of Therapeutic Touch lies in the intelligent direction of significant life energies from the person playing the role of healer to the healee (the ill person).

There are many theories about this healer-healee interaction which we shall discuss in a later chapter; however, since speculations about the dynamics of the healing act without providing an experiential base can result in mere intellectual exercise, I would like to share some structured experiences with you first. In these exercises, you will be immediately exposed to a sizable range of energetics similar to those you will be experiencing during the process of Therapeutic Touch.

These exercises are fun. They are simple and can be done either by yourself or with others. Any equipment you will need can be found around the house or inexpensively purchased. Let us begin.

THERAPEUTIC TOUCH SELF-KNOWLEDGE TEST #1: YOU DO NOT STOP AT YOUR SKIN

The first experiential knowing which I'd like to share with you is that you can be consciously aware of a flow of energy in the "empty" space beyond the skin boundaries of your hands. It is very useful to capture first-time experiences as they happen, so, as you do these exercises, keep a pad and pencil handy so that you can take notes for later review.

1. The first step is to sit comfortably with both feet on the ground and simply place your hands so that the palms face each other. Hold your elbows away from the trunk of your body and do not rest your lower arms in your lap. Now bring your palms as close together as you can get them without having them touch each other, so that they are perhaps one-eighth to one-quarter inch apart (see Figure 1).
2. The next step is to separate the palms of your hands by about two inches and then slowly bring them back to their original position, about one-eighth to one-quarter inch apart from one another.
3. Now separate your palms by about four inches and, again, slowly bring them back to their original position, as noted above.

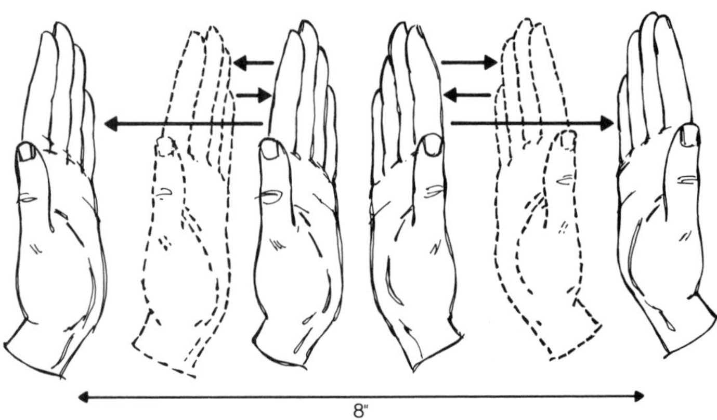

Figure 1. Bring hands as close together as you can without the palms touching each other. Then bring hands apart about two inches. Return hands slowly to original position. Repeat, however, each time separate the palms by an additional two inches, until they are finally eight inches apart.

4. Repeat this procedure. However, this time, separate your palms by about six inches. Keep your motions slow and steady. As you return your hands to their original position, notice if you begin to feel a build-up of pressure between your hands or if you feel any other significant sensation.
5. Once again separate your palms, this time until they are about eight inches apart. Do not immediately return your hands to their original position. Instead, as you bring your hands close together, at about every two inches, experience the pressure field you have built up by stopping for a moment and slowly trying to compress the field between your hands (see Figure 2). You may experience this as a "bouncy" feeling.
6. Spend the next full minute in experiencing this field between your hands and try to determine what other characteristics of the field you feel besides the pressure and the bounciness or elasticity. At the end of the time, write down these other characteristics on a piece of paper before you go on to the next paragraph, and then draw a line under your last entry.

What characteristics of the field did you find besides the sense of pressure and the bounciness?

Some of the field characteristics other students have found are sensations of heat, cold, and tingling and a sense of pulsations. However, do

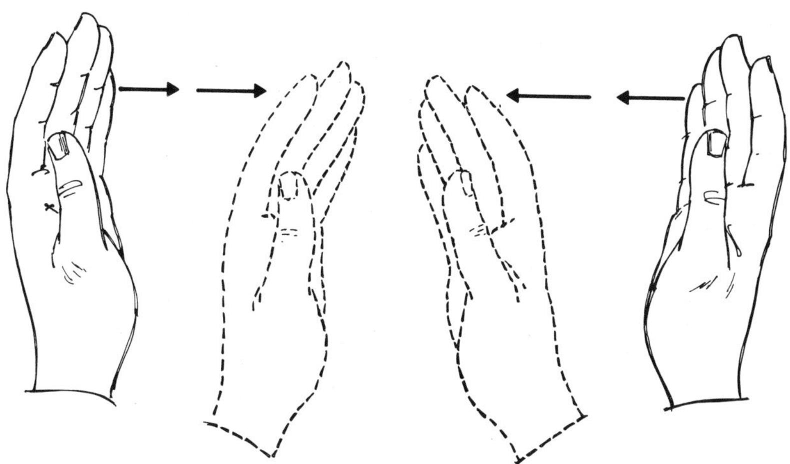

Figure 2. When the hands are about eight inches apart, slowly bring them together. At every two inches test the field between your hands for a sense of bounciness or elasticity.

not accept their experiences; experiment for yourself and determine what, if any, reality this experience has for *you.*

I cannot stress this last statement too strongly, for you will find that at every phase of the Therapeutic Touch process it is *your* sense of the reality of the situation that will be the sounding board for your therapeutic intervention. Teach yourself now to develop confidence in your own reality, that is, what it is that appears to you to be the truth about your own experiences.

This exercise is used in many cultures for many reasons. Most frequently, it is used as an exercise in concentration; however, I like to use it for additional reasons as well. Interestingly, you will find that the impressions you have just experienced are very similar to the cues you will pick up from the healee's field during Therapeutic Touch. These cues, with the development of expertise, will be an important foundation upon which you will subsequently base the course of your conscious and knowledgeable intervention.

The second reason I like to use this exercise to test the notion that you do not stop at your skin is that you can do it anywhere and at any time—I hardly need to point out, I am sure, that you take your hands wherever you go! It is a most important reason, however, for in practicing this exercise on yourself you gain a kind of self-knowledge which you can test for reliability.

THERAPEUTIC TOUCH SELF-KNOWLEDGE TEST #2: USING YOUR FIELD AS A DATA BASE

Now that you have had one experiential base for recognizing that the energies of your personal life field extend beyond your skin boundaries, what other information can you elicit from that extension of yourself?

The next two exercises work best if they are done in group settings. For the purposes of this exercise, have the members of the group sit next to each other in a circle. If they have never done the previous exercise, teach it to them. After they have experienced that exercise, each of you should do the following:

1. Sit comfortably. If you are sitting in a chair, have both feet on the floor. For the purposes of this exercise, you might like to

close your eyes lightly; however, it is not necessary. Have a pad or piece of paper and a pencil within easy reach. Whatever you will write will be primarily for your own information, and there is no need for you to share this with anyone unless you would like to do so. Therfore, write as fully as you wish for the purposes of your own self-learning at a later date.

2. In the previous exercise, you learned that you did not stop at your skin. Knowing that, for one minute, in your mind's eye explore the area just beyond your right shoulder and try to get an idea of what that space "feels" like.
3. As you get a sense of that personal space, tuck that information in your memory to be recalled later.
4. Now, "extend" that space beyond your right shoulder so that it reaches toward your neighbor on your right hand side. Do not exert any physical effort. Direct the energy in that space effortlessly towards your neighbor.
5. It may happen that various impressions may arise in your mind. They may be colors, pictorial visualizations, symbols, words, feelings, or sensations that may or may not have meaning for you. Simply be a spectator to this display and tuck whatever information arises into your memory.
6. Do this for one full minute and then write down your impressions as clearly as you can remember them. When you have finished, draw a line across the page under your last impression and go on to the next exercise.

THERAPEUTIC TOUCH SELF-KNOWLEDGE TEST #3: INTENSIFYING THE FIELD EFFECTS

For the next exercise, you and each member of your group will need a piece of absorbent cotton that is cut a bit larger than the size of the hand. Rolls of unsterilized absorbent cotton can be purchased in most drug or general stores. One small box can be used for several people. Have the group members remain seated as they were in the circle; each member's piece of paper and pencil should remain within easy reach.

1. Each person should lay the piece of cotton on her/his hand.
2. Then place the other hand over the cotton pad without touching it (see Figure 3).
3. Become aware of the field—your personal space—just beyond the palm of your uppermost hand.
4. Using that field awareness, try to visualize reaching down with that hand's field to the hand that is lying under the cotton pad.
5. As you did in Therapeutic Touch Self-knowledge Test #2, move the hands slowly and steadily nearer and then farther away from each other. Keep your hand movements within an eight-inch radius of each other. Do this for one full minute and note down the feelings that you experience in your hands. Write them down and draw a line under the last entry. These feelings will be similar to the heat, cold, tingling, pressure, pulsations, and so on that you felt in the previous exercise, but they will be more clearly and strongly felt. Continue now to the next part of this exercise.
6. Now, have each person in the group give his or her piece of cotton to the person on his or her left. Each person will receive a piece of cotton from his or her right hand neighbor.
7. Each person should now lay the piece of transferred cotton on his or her hand as before and place the other hand over, but not touching, the cotton. Now, use the field of the overlying hand to "reach" down to the hand under the cotton pad; that is, feel as though you were reaching down from the hand above

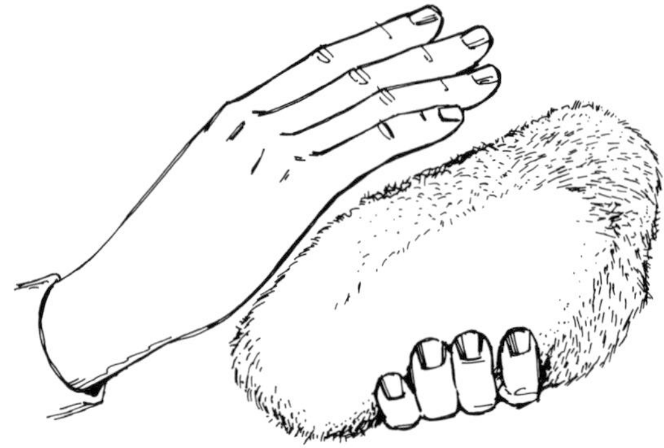

Figure 3. Place other hand over cotton pad without touching it.

the cotton pad to the hand on which the pad rests, but do not touch your hands together.

8. Now, keeping the overlying hand within an eight-inch radius of the cotton pad, slowly move this hand closer and then away from the cotton and become aware of any impressions that arise in your mind. Either tuck these impressions in your memory or write them on the piece of paper in front of you as the thoughts arise. Do this exercise for a full two minutes.

   Do not question the impressions, no matter how illogical, odd, or unfamiliar they may seem. Simply accept them and record them. You may have impressions of colors, pictorial visualizations, symbols, words, feelings, or sensations which may or may not hold meaning for you. Quietly be aware of whatever arises in your mind for the next two minutes and record it.

9. Take one final half-minute to complete any impressions you jotted down or to add any connecting or clarifying phrases.

10. Scan the four groups of notes you wrote and analyze them for similarities and for differences. The first and third entries will be concerned with yourself, and the second and fourth entries will be related to your interactions with the field of your right hand neighbor.

11. As noted above, the information you have gathered is primarily for your own learning, and there is no need to share this material with the group members. However, should you wish to share this material, ask the permission of the person sitting on your right before you tell of your second and fourth groups of impressions. Most people will willingly give you this permission; however, it might be considered an invasion of privacy, which is understandable.

    While people are talking about their experiences, it will be most useful if the original owner of the cotton does not give a trace of a hint, either verbally or nonverbally, to the person speaking about her cotton. Adhere to this convention until all persons in the circle who wish to tell of their impressions have had a chance to do so.

12. Now, the persons who have been talked about will have their opportunity to tell the group whether the persons holding their original pieces of cotton were correct in their impressions.

The number of "hits" will be surprising, I am quite sure; however, do not disregard the "misses." These should be examined for personal meaning. Also, an interesting occurrence that sometimes happens is that a person wrapped up in the intensity of the exercise may "leap-frog" beyond the person sitting next to him or her and inadvertently pick up correct impressions of someone else in the room. Search out this possibility and, if it has occurred, see if you can figure out why and how it happened.

All of the exercises suggested above are simulations of experiences that you will have while doing Therapeutic Touch, and, therefore, they should be practiced, thought about, and, if possible, discussed with others of like interests. I shall refer to these practices as we go along in this book, so that we shall have a commonality of experience as a basis for discussing the actual techniques of Therapeutic Touch.

So far, in these exercises, we have found out that:

1. You do not stop at your skin; there is a field beyond your skin boundaries which can be experienced.
2. You can use this field as a data base; when you turn your attention to this personal space, you find that it does help you to elicit additional cues about your environment.
3. You can intensify these field effects so that they are more perceptible to you.

This is quite a tidy bit of information; however, is this the most that we can say about this field—that it is somewhere "out there"? I think we can do better than that; I think we can demonstrate that this field has a physically perceivable pattern. At this writing, this pattern has been demonstrated in approximately 80% of the several hundreds of persons upon whom the following exercise has been tried.

It should be noted that, unlike the previous exercises, this demonstration is *not* at all related to healing in any way—as far as I am presently aware. As you will see, a kind of dowsing rod will be used to demonstrate this field pattern; however, I know little about dowsing and probably do not use these rods within any context related to dowsing. What intrigues me is the patterning that I have found to be an invariant, or constant, in 80% of persons. I do not have any idea or theory about why the rods assume these patterns when they are used as described below. Try it and see what you make of it.

THERAPEUTIC TOUCH SELF-KNOWLEDGE TEST #4: THERE IS A PERCEIVABLE PATTERNING IN THE HUMAN FIELD

For this test, you will need someone on whom you can demonstrate, and you will also need the following objects: two metal clothes hangers, a pair of pliers or a wire cutter, two 3″ X 5″ cardboard filing cards, and six one-half inch pieces of cellophane tape.

1. Cut both wire hangers at *A* and *B* as shown in Figure 4.
2. Straighten out each cut hanger so that the side and bottom wires are at ninety degree angles to one another, as shown in Figure 5.
3. Take the two 3″ X 5″ filing cards and roll each card along its longer side. Now tape the free ends so that you have two five-inch cylinders, as shown in Figure 6.
4. Slip the cylinders onto the shorter arm of each of the cut hangers and then bend the tips of these arms to hold the cylinders in place, as shown in Figure 7.
5. Now, have your companion lie on his or her back with his or her hands at his or her sides in a relaxed, comfortable position.
6. Pick up the rods and place your hands over the cardboard cylinders. Do not squeeze the cylinders; the cylinders are meant to keep the rods free from any pressure you might inadvertently try to exert on the rods. Hold the rods lightly in front of you

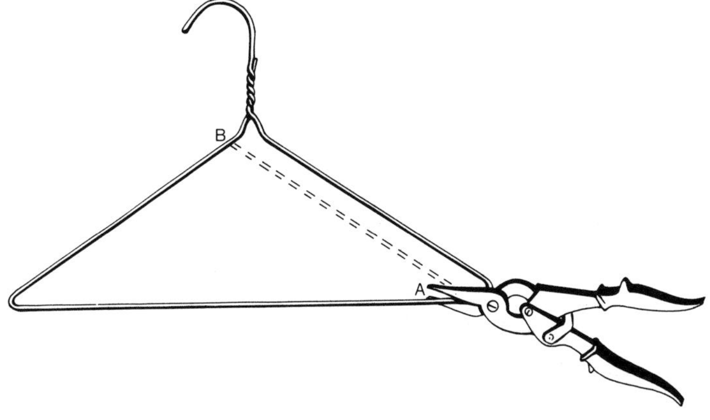

Figure 4. Cut wire hanger at A ***and*** B.

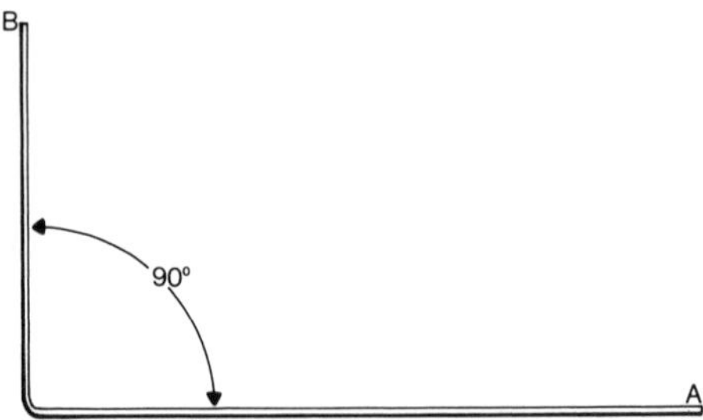

Figure 5. Straighten the cut hanger so that the side and bottom wires are at a 90° angle to each.

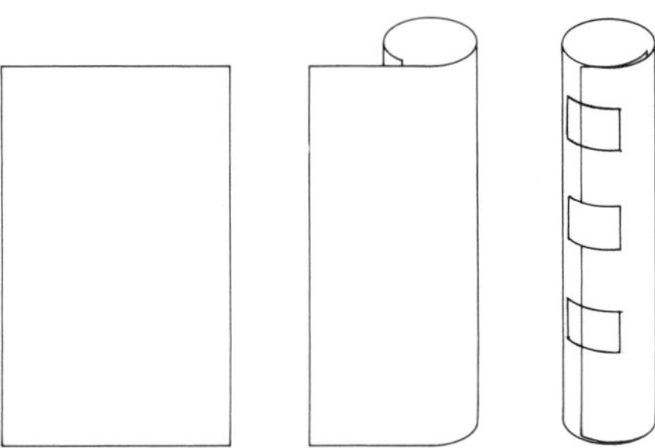

Figure 6. Take two three-inch cardboard filing cards and roll each card along its longer side. Tape the free ends so that you have two five-inch cylinders.

Figure 7. Slip one cylinder onto the shorter arm of each of the cut hangers; then bend the tip of the short arms to hold the cylinders in place.

with your arms slightly extended, so that your elbows do not rest on the trunk of your body. The long arms of the rods should point directly in front of you.

7. The rods will move freely in the cylinders. This movement is mostly due to the gravitational field. In order to prevent this movement, the long arms of the rods must be kept parallel

to the floor; if you dip them, they will respond to the g-field and start to circle again. This will necessitate your keeping your eyes on the rods to make sure that they don't dip. If there is a third person available, that person can also watch the rods and check you.

Admittedly, this is a makeshift affair that I devised. What I sometimes do, in order to assure that any inadvertent dipping of the rods will be noticed, is to take two large, empty gelatin capsules (such as those which contain vitamins) and carefully open each of them. I then partly fill each capsule with water and reclose the capsules. I now glue one of the capsules to the long arm of each rod. The water in the capsule will act as a level to further assure that you will keep the rods parallel to the floor, and they will not interfere with the demonstration.

As long as the rods are kept free to move without undo interference, the pattern that I have found to occur in 80% of people is that these rods will cross over each other (or point at each other, if the hands are held too far apart) over five specific parts of the body. These five parts of the body are: the forehead, the throat, the physiological solar plexus (about two to three inches below the bottom of the sternum, or middle of the rib cage), the knees, and the ankles. The rods will not react while over the other areas of the body.

8. Holding onto the rods as described above, stand about one foot beyond the head of your companion. Unless you have by some chance happened upon an electrical circuit or water pipes under the flooring, the rods will be straight out in front of you.

9. Now, keeping your hands and therefore the rods in the same position, slowly and steadily move along the side of your companion toward his or her feet, remembering to keep the long arms of the rods parallel to the floor.

10. As you move down the side of your partner, note whether the rods cross each other over the areas noted above: the forehead, the throat, the physiological solar plexus, the knees, and the ankles.

In any large sample, the rods will cross, I am by now quite sure, four-fifths of the time. I do not know why this happens, but it will occur reliably even at some distance from the body; for example, if the subject is lying on the floor and the person

> handling the rods is standing and is an adult, there is usually about three and one-half to four feet separating the rods from the subject's body surface.

There is much that I do not understand about this strange occurrence; however, what impresses me—and I therefore offer it to you for your own speculation—is that somehow there is an interaction occurring in the "empty" space between two people who are engaged as noted above and that such patterning can be reliably predicted eighty percent of the time. That is a neat confidence level; it gives me confidence to feel assured that there is something "out there," that indeed I don't stop at my skin, and, if this is so, that I can consciously and intelligently learn to use this natural extension of myself both for a more complete understanding of myself and also, through that understanding, for the well-being of others.

4

Centering: The "Effortless Effort"

Therapeutic Touch is basically a healing meditation; that is, the primary act is to center oneself in a natural, tension-free manner and to maintain that center throughout the entirety of the Therapeutic Touch process.

There are four phases to Therapeutic Touch, and each phase will be discussed in one of the following chapters. Specifically, these phases are:

1. Centering oneself physically and psychologically; that is, finding within oneself an inner reference of stability.
2. Exercising the natural sensitivity of the hand to assess the energy field of the healee for cues to differences in the quality of energy flow.

3. Mobilizing areas in the healee's energy field that the healer may perceive as being non-flowing; that is, sluggish, congested, or static.
4. The conscious direction by the healer of his or her excess body energies to assist the healee to repattern his or her own energies.

This last phase in particular may seem strangely worded to the reader unaccustomed to thinking in terms of bioenergetics and psychoenergetics; however, the writer asks their indulgence at this time, for a more thorough discussion will be given in later chapters. Moreover, although these stages are stated sequentially, the reader will note, once he or she progresses in the practice of Therapeutic Touch, that in fact a certain simultaneity may occur. I do not know why this occurs, but it can be conceived that from the moment one turns one's attention to helping or healing another, an energetic interchange between those two people has already begun. For instance, even during the assessment it appears that the healer actually begins to transfer energy to the healee, perhaps due to the automaticity that seems to underlie the natural dynamics of interchange that marks human relationships. You, as healer, are interested in determining the best way to help the healee, and so during the assessment you focus your attention on the healee with this in mind. The focusing of your intention gives explicit, although perhaps unconscious, direction to your energy flow. On the other hand, in the close and highly personalized interaction that is coupled to the transfer of energy from healer to healee during the fourth phase, you will find that certain as yet poorly understood factors within yourself become aware of fuller data about the healee's condition. It is the validity of this personal knowledge that each must explore for him- or herself to qualify the spectrum of reality in which he or she is engaged during this healing act.

Centering refers to a sense of self-relatedness that can be thought of as a place of inner being, a place of quietude within oneself where one can feel truly integrated, unified, and focused. It has been described as the source of our conscious awareness of our involvement in life; however, it is a personal space apart from either the involvement or the consequent reaction to that involvement. Although it is structured, in the sense that one must consciously direct one's energies in order to become aware of that space within, the act of centering does not involve an exertion of effort, a straining of what I call "the muscles of the brain." A beetling of brows or a holding of breath will not get you there; centering is a conscious direction of attention inwards, an "effortless effort" that is conceptual but that can also be experiential.

Peper, after studying the writer while she was doing Therapeutic Touch to ill persons and then replicating that study with other persons who also played the role of healer at a later date, calls Therapeutic Touch "a healing meditation." (see Appendix II). This description was based on physiological data recorded via electroencephalography, electromyography, and electrooculography during Therapeutic Touch and then compared to similar data derived from research on the meditative process. It would seem that this similarity could be based on the centrality of centering to the helping or healing act in Therapeutic Touch. As noted above, the first thing one does in Therapeutic Touch is to center and, ideally, the person playing the role of healer stays on center throughout the entirety of the process; and, if he or she strays from that state of consciousness, he or she returns to center once she is aware of the delinquency. It is because of this conscious effortless effort to remain in this unitive state that I sometimes refer to Therapeutic Touch as a yoga of healing. As one learns to maintain this state of centeredness for a few consecutive minutes, a concomitant feeling of confidence encourages the individual to begin to explore this personal space. The experience brings to cognition facets of oneself that have previously lain latent—facets that, as one repeats the experience, become increasingly actualized.

This act of centering happens to be one of the touchstones of creativity. Concomitant with this process, therefore, an insight into one's self might arise to consciousness. Other innovative approaches to life experience may also occur as the person begins to recognize ordering principles within the microcosm of one's own dynamics.

Experience and studies I have done indicate that this goal does not come easily, however. It does not seem to be enough that the person who wishes to play the role of healer simply *wants* to heal—if this were so, surely every parent who wanted to help his or her sick child could do so. This, of course, is not the case. Based on several studies over the past eight years, it seems that there are at least three conditions which have to be met for a person to become a really helpful healer. They are:

1. Intentionality.
2. Motivation in the interests of the healee.
3. Not only an ability to confront oneself, but also the willingness to do so.

The reasons for these conclusions are several. Intentionality carries the connotation that in the intentional act one has a goal in view; that is, the healer knows what he or she is going to do. Anyone who intervenes in another's health care should do so from a knowledgeable base; the intervention should be intelligent, and the intervenor—the healer in this case—should understand the process in which he or she is involved. In other words, the healer should have a goal, a plan of action for his or her engagement with the healee. The requisite that the healer's motivation be in the interests of the healee, rather than motivated by the needs of his or her own ego structure, is based on recognizing that psychodynamically the energy wrapped up in the emotions is directional. That is, emotions concern feelings about something. Therefore motivation, which provides the context for the working out of the emotion, nourishes and guides that directionality. Finally, the act of healing is a power tool, and the person who wishes to play the role of healer must understand, at the least, *why* he or she wants to do it—that is, at the minimum, the healer must be able to confront him- or herself on at least one question: Why do I want to be healer? In a sense, it does not matter what the answer is, but each individual must acknowledge the answer.

The act of centering can be entered at many different levels. Let us begin to capture, describe, and understand the experience just as it occurs; that is, let us take a phenomenonological approach and become aware of gestures, bodily sensations, inward feelings, and emerging ideas that occur to consciousness in the act of centering. For the purposes of discussion, I am now going to try to record the beginning experiences that occur as I try to center.

I am sitting on the floor, and I've just crossed my legs in a half-lotus position—painfully! I get myself into position, lay one hand on the other, gently rock my body from side to side an inch or two to put my body in alignment with my center of gravity, and then I lean my body backwards slightly, about one or two inches. I find that I am now in a very stable position.

I close my eyes and take several deep breaths. I relax the muscles at the back of my neck and check that my extremities are relaxed. I feel comfortable. My body feels at ease. If I feel any sense of tension, I release it, just let it go. I seem to search out physiological tensions as well as bodily tensions and release my awareness of them.

I am aware of a rhythmic synchronization to my respirations, of breathing deeply, slowly, and easily. I also feel as though the vibrations indicative of my being are more rhythmical, more integrated.

I am aware that the back of my hands fit neatly into the hollow of the arch of my uppermost foot, which is up-turned on my thigh. I feel all together in my space.

I am aware of energy flowing between my shoulders and in the back of my neck. It is a vital, but comfortable feeling, and a sense of quietude prevails.

I try to go more deeply within my consciousness. This directing of thought does not disturb me. The feeling of boundless quietude continues. I feel as though I have all my faculties at my command, and I am enjoying a unitive sense of physical and psychological attunement and well-being.

These behaviors seem to be the process by which I center physically and psychodynamically. Let me now try to translate this description into specific instructions for the reader who would like to replicate the experience at these levels and add to it his or her own unique behaviors.

THERAPEUTIC TOUCH SELF-KNOWLEDGE TEST #5: PHYSICAL AND PSYCHOLOGICAL ASPECTS OF CENTERING

1. Sit in a relaxed position, either in a chair or on the floor, so that your body is in alignment.
2. Either lay your hands comfortably on your lap, if you are sitting on a chair, or fold your hands one on top the other if you are sitting on the floor or ground with your legs crossed.
3. Slowly move your body one to two inches from side to side two or three times so that when you stop you feel as though your spine is in postural alignment.
4. Now tilt your body back about one to two inches. This should be a comfortable position; your vertebrae should be aligned so that they easily carry the weight of your body.
5. Close your eyes and breathe slowly, evenly, and effortlessly.
6. Feel out—that is, become aware of—your tensions and purposefully relax them. This may be easiest to do upon exhalation.
7. Feel your body to be in balance.
8. Go more deeply within your consciousness. At each deeper level of consciousness, be aware of any tension and release that tension.

9. When you have attained a sense of inner equilibrium, you should feel that you can call upon your physical and psychodynamic energies on command and direct them as you wish—that is, you should feel that you are both aware and in control of your own dynamics.

This is an elementary method for experiencing the act of centering one's consciousness. There are many methods of centering that are taught as part of meditative practices, as methods of awareness, or in prayer.[1] Whichever method one feels most at ease with will invariably work well with Therapeutic Touch.

Some people use the recollection of a personal image or a symbol to help them center. Others use repetitive sound, such as the intoning of a mantra—that is, a word of power. According to Benson, this word may be meaningless.[2] For example, one of the words he suggests is the repetition of the word "one." An amusing story has it that when a well-known Eastern religious teacher was told what Benson suggested, he replied, "Well, there is no need even to say, 'One, one, one, one. . . .' If one is in the right frame of mind, all one need do is repeat: 'Coco-cola, coco-cola, coco-cola! . . .'"

From my own experience, I find that it is useful to teach in the most simple way, not necessarily to make the task easy, but because there is frequently a certain elegance in the simple way that can carry a pithy and sometimes profound message. Because of this, I would like to suggest another method of capturing the experience of centering, one which I find to be of particular help for people just learning how to center. The future rememberance of this experience will help one to come to center almost immediately.

THERAPEUTIC TOUCH SELF-KNOWLEDGE TEST #6: INSTANT CENTERING

1. Sit comfortably, but in postural alignment, while doing this Test.
2. Relax. To assure this, I suggest that you check out your favorite

[1] Patricia Carrington, *Freedom in Meditation* (Garden City, N.Y.: Anchor Press/Doubleday, 1978), pp. 20–36.

[2] Herbert Benson, *The Relaxation Response* (N.Y.: Morrow, 1975).

tension spots and relax those areas of your body. If your neck or shoulder muscles are in tension, strongly depress your shoulders—that is, push your shoulders down so that they are not hunched up toward your neck.

3. Inhale deeply and gently.
4. Slowly exhale.
5. Inhale again—and there you are! It is just here, in this state between breaths which you are now experiencing, that a state similar to the centering experience can be simulated. It is this state of balance, of equipoise, and of quietude that marks the experience of centering.

I like this exercise for several reasons. Primarily, I like it because of its similarity to the actual experience of centering. However, I also like it because once you have done it, you needn't ever do it again in that way. The human mind has a wonderful capacity to recall not only an experience but even the atmosphere or emotional tone surrounding a meaningful occurrence in one's life. Therefore, before one begins Therapeutic Touch, a recollection of this experience of centering can be recalled to mind instantly, and the individual can learn to simulate that state of awareness upon self-command.

The ability to recapture the state of this centering of consciousness instantaneously is very useful because, as noted above, in Therapeutic Touch the healer always tries to operate from center. One finds that in so doing the person on center feels securely in control both of his or her energies and of the direction of his or her attention. Moreover, being on center tends to put events into a rational perspective devoid of personal attachments or biases. The person on center acts from the surety of his or her own frame of reference and, therefore, does not easily fall into one of the major traps of the highly personalized interaction involved in the healing act, that of a too personal identification with the difficulties of the patient. To open oneself in this way may bring in its train the possibility of allowing oneself to become part of the problem—and then one has to face the question: Who will heal the healer?

5

The Assessment: Appreciation of the Field Characteristics of the Individual Healee

Therapeutic Touch is foremost a conscious act of therapeutic intervention. Although it is concerned with subtle energies, their direction and modulation are based upon as much information as the person playing the role of healer can command and, to that extent, Therapeutic Touch is a knowledgeable intervention. This base of information rests upon data gathered in the second phase of Therapeutic Touch, which is called, for convenience sake, the Assessment.

The Assessment derives from the motivation of the healer to meet the needs of the healee, a major condition for results in the best interests of the healee, as was noted in the previous chapter. Since he or she really wishes to help the individual, the healer will use any means available in order to do this intelligently. Of foremost importance is the bringing forward of all recollectable information about human function that one has gathered during his or her past experience and education. Therapeutic Touch is not a miracle; it is a natural potential that can be actualized under the appropriate circumstances, and one of the circumstances is that the healer intervene from a knowledgeable base.

Although much of this knowledge is based on facets of ourselves which we are not ordinarily aware of in our usual activities of daily living, there is much that our more common senses can tell us, and, in the best interests of our healees, we should not overlook this knowledge.

For this reason, I would recommend that you begin to make note of the ill person from your first contact. If the contact is by phone, note the person's voice: What does it tell you about the tonal qualities of his personality? For example, what does his voice tell you about his emotional level, his anxieties, his fears? Should your first encounter be on sight, quietly and unobtrusively search his physical activities for aids to understanding his illness. Notice how he walks as he comes into the room: Is there hesitancy in his gait? Does he seem to be in balance? Does he favor one side of his body during locomotion? Notice his postural stance: Is there any guarding of parts of his body? Are his shoulders hunched up in tension? Be aware of any facial signs of emotional involvement as he sits down.

Observations such as these can be invaluable as information sources, and so it will be worth your while to compose for yourself a list of behaviors to watch for from the time the healee enters the room until he sits down near you. A very useful way to gain experience in gathering this kind of information is to visit an out-patient department of a nearby large hospital and keep an account of your observations of people as they enter the door. If you want to check your observations, as a rule, casual conversations are easy to start in the waiting rooms of most out-patient clinics, for most people will welcome an opportunity to relieve the boredom of the usual long wait, particularly if they are able to talk about themselves!

Besides this telereceptive way of gaining information about a person's condition, Therapeutic Touch uses information available from the personal field of an individual. I am not using the term "field" in a mysterious way; I am talking about a human field as a biophysical fact. By this I refer to the common knowledge that the human body's functions, such as locomotion, occur via the electrical conductance that occurs throughout the neuromuscular system, and that one of the basic principles in biophysics recognizes that in all cases of electrical conductance, there must be a field to carry the charge. One of the first people to demonstrate that field forces exist not only in but also outside the nerve during excitation was Harold Saxon Burr and his coworkers at the Yale University School of Medicine.[1] This unusual man spent more than forty years of his life in painstaking studies to map and measure the parameters of what he came to call "the fields of life." Among his findings were that concomitant alterations occur in these fields of life, or L-fields, according to the physical and mental condition of the individual subject, and that these changes in the L-field are so reliable that they can be used in the diagnosis of various disorders.

I think that humans can become aware of fields such as the L-fields (for there is more than one field that humans are subject to). Note, for instance, the effect of a field with which you are interacting, although it usually goes unnoticed, as you sit in your chair to read this book—the gravitational fields which acts to hold you in that chair. I would like to suggest some simple ways in which you can find this out for yourself.

The way I get some sense of the irregularities in an individual's field that may be related to his illness is by a process based, again, on as much common sense data as are available to me. In order to do this, I started by reading the literature and searching out descriptions by healers all over the world on how they determine a person's illness. First of all, they refer to the area surrounding a person, rather than to the physical body itself. I find it very interesting that their verbal descriptions of this field's characteristics are rather limited, regardless of what culture they come from; in fact, there are only about a half-dozen ways they phrase these descriptions. Healers say they feel "heat," "cold," "tingling," "pressure," "electric shocks," "pulsations," or, occasionally, some other sensation. Because of this universality of expression, I think these terms indicate a common experience for which we do not as yet have an adequately expressive language. Nevertheless, I accept the words as a true explanation of the subjective experience, and I go on to note that the expression most often used refers to temperature differential. I then ask myself: How does one feel differences in temperature? Of course, we feel temperature differences relative to the ambient temperature. I, therefore, actually note the temperature in the room with my hand, feeling both for the temperature of the room and for any breeze there may be or

[1] Harold S. Burr, *The Fields of Life* (NY: Ballantine, 1973).

for any sense of humidity, and I use these environmental data as a base for whatever temperature I experience as I bring my hands within about two inches of the healee's skin surface.

I use one other clue, based upon my knowledge that human beings are bilaterally symmetrical. Using this recognized fact as a base, I realize that if I feel a particular temperature on the right side of a person's field, I should also feel the same temperature on the left side. If I do not find this to be so, I simply recognize that there is a difference.

Basing my assessment of someone's condition on the above information, I now do the following after I have approached the individual and have centered myself.

THERAPEUTIC TOUCH SELF-KNOWLEDGE TEST #7: THE ASSESSMENT

1. Remembering from Therapeutic Touch Self-knowledge Test #1 (see Chapter 3) that I "do not stop at my skin," I place my hands two to three inches from the person's skin. It does not matter where I begin; however, it seems to work out naturally to start at the head, since the ill person is either sitting or lying down and the healer is either standing up or sitting down. As one reaches out one's hand from either position, the hand level easily reaches the head of the healee.
2. Stand in front of the healee with the hands outstretched towards his or her head, two to three inches from his or her skin surface, and test the left side area against the right side area. Move your hands slowly but steadily down from his or her head area to his or her face area, all the while keeping yourself sensitive to any sign of temperature change in your hands. The timing to scan from the top of the head to the chin should be within the range of seven to ten seconds. Do not linger, asking yourself: "Did I feel something or didn't I feel something?" It is very easy to mix oneself up when beginning; therefore, force yourself to move on within the suggested time frame. If you have questions, you can recheck the area after you have done a complete head to toe assessment.

3. Continue in this manner to scan the entire front of the body, tucking any information you receive in the back of your head for the time being.
4. When you have finished the front of the person, do the same thing to the back of the person. Again, start at the head and go down the person's body. You will find that your brain will reward consistency in input of information by bringing to mind relevant associated ideas as you scan. Try to keep track of all the data until you have finished the scan.
5. When you have completely finished the scan, go back to any areas about which you had doubts and recheck your impressions.

You may find that instead of relating to a temperature differential as you scan, you are relating to one of the other sensations noted above: tingling, pressure, electric shock, or pulsation. Keep track of these clues as they occur in the same manner noted for temperature changes.

Although we do not recognize it in our culture, other cultures recognize several energy centers in the body. In the East, two of these energy centers are recognized to be in the palms of the hands. If you turn your hand palm up, you will notice that the center of the palm is depressed. This well or depression in the center of the palm is considered to be the physical locus for these hand energy centers (called *chakras* in Sanskrit). From my reading of the literature of the Aruvedic medicine of India, it seems to me that it is these *chakras,* one in each hand, that are the functional agents in all therapeutic uses of hands. These, however, are only secondary *chakras.* The primary ones, relate to the endocrine glands as physical loci.[2] The Aruvedic literature describes these *chakras* as agents for the transforming of universal energies, as they become available to our bodies, to levels which can be used by human beings. Within this paradigm, the energies enter through some counterpart of the spleen which Western science has not as yet recognized. From the spleenic area, the energies disperse in five major streams to energize the various critical parts of the body in different combinations of the five streams. Interestingly, after these energies have circuited the body, they enter the arms. When they reach "the knot of the wrist," however, they reconstitute themselves and exit through the five fingers in their original state, that of the five major streams.

[2]Charles W. Leadbeater, *The Chakras* (Wheaton, Illinois: Theosophical Publishing House, 1940).

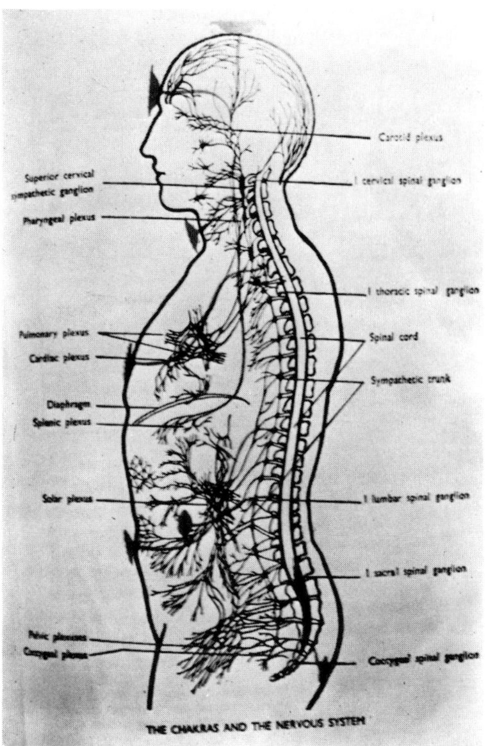

Chakras in juxtaposition to the human nervous system (photo—courtesy of The Theosophical Publishing House, Madras, India).

Although these conceptions seem strange to us in the West, I often have cause to recognize that the reality of the East, although built upon subjective experience rather than upon the objective evidence considered the basis of reality in the West, has as much reliability in its own right as does our Western reality. For instance, the most respected treatises on yoga, which is one of the six Indian orthodox systems of philosophy, are *The Yoga Sutras of Patanjali.* The time of writing of these commentaries is controversial; however, they are thought to have been written about the second century A.D. The commentaries are made up of aphorisms that say: If you do this and that, such and such will happen. It speaks to the reliability of this information to know that today, 1,700 years after Patanjali wrote his commentaries based upon life experience, if one reads his book and does this and that, one will indeed find that such and such will still happen.

In exercising my abilities to do the Assessment, I found this advice from my teacher, Ms. Kunz, about whom I've written above, to be most useful: Use every means to test the validity of your perceptions. You are,

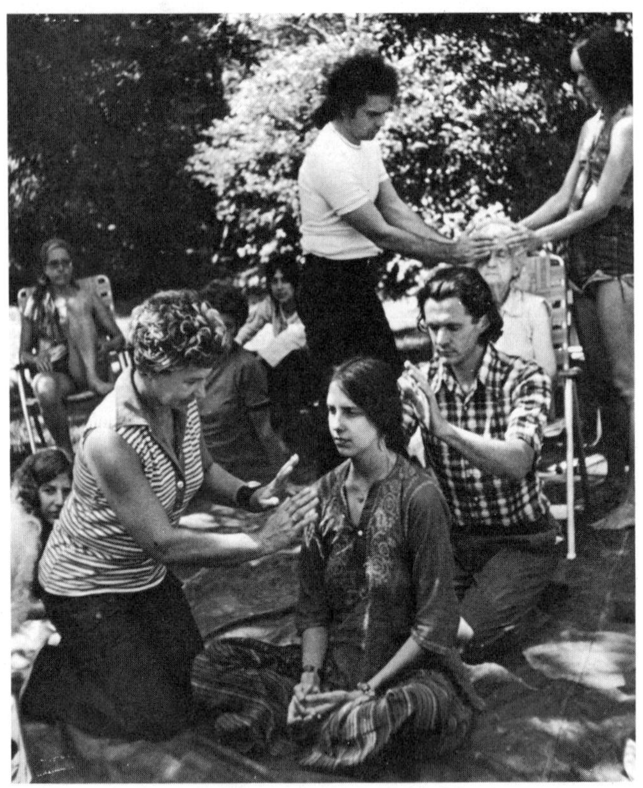

Therapeutic Touch in teams.

first of all, learning to use these latent abilities: Do not be afraid to make a mistake. Your beginning attempts will be in accord with the laws of probability; and if you admit that you are a beginner, this is an acceptable recognition. If you give yourself to a serious study of Therapeutic Touch, however, you will find that your natural abilities will be honed to a fine edge with frequent practice; and, in a surprisingly short time, you will find that you can use your Assessment with as much reliability as you use any other evaluative tool.

One objective method by which you can test yourself is to write down your assessment of the individual's energy distribution before you find out the healee's diagnosis. If you do not have writing facilities at hand, tell your assessment to someone—not to your best friend, who too frequently will agree with you that you said something that will turn out to be similar to a verified diagnosis. Rather choose an impersonal observer, someone who is not close to you, someone who can objectively gauge whether your assessment agrees with the facts of the case. If you are right, the reliability of your ability to assess will be reinforced; if your assessment turns out to be wrong, you now have an immediate opportunity to learn from your mistakes.

It should be clearly recognized that what you are doing in the Assessment has no relation to other types of evaluation, such as medical diagnosis. In this type of Assessment, you are sensitizing yourself to sense changes in energy flow; if you note a difference, you are simply saying to yourself, as you scan the healee's field, "Here, there is a difference." If you make mental connections about the possible meaning of the differences in energy flow that you feel, which may be based on your collateral knowledge of anatomy, physiology, or neurology, then that is splendid; but that is not needed in the Assessment as it is outlined above. As noted, in the Assessment, you are only looking for differences in energy flow. Every facet of Therapeutic Touch is concerned with energy flow, as a matter of fact; from this point of view, one can therefore see that a medical diagnosis would be highly inappropriate, since medical diagnoses arise out of a classification system that is unlike the perceptions we are

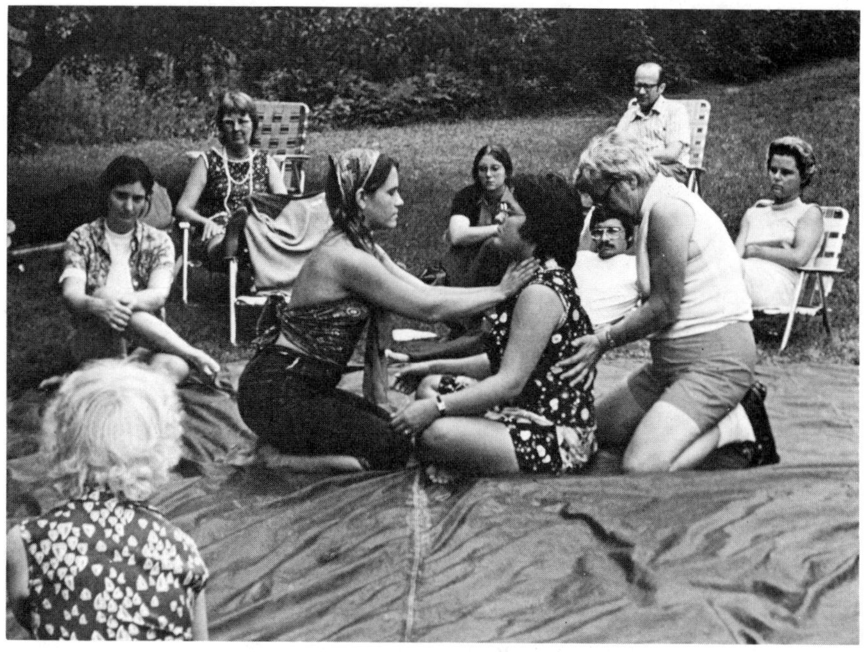

Therapeutic Touch in teams.

dealing with. The perceptions that we are dealing with in Therapeutic Touch are at a very direct, perhaps primitive, level. Medical diagnosis, on the other hand, is based upon a very complex system of classification that is quite sophisticated, and so there is little relation between the two; indeed, there is little reason why there should be, or why there need be.

There are a number of ways one can increase the sensitivity of the hand to perceive changes in the personal field of the healee. One that is used, sometimes quite instinctively, is to place the palms of the hands in front of you and then to rub them briskly together. Within a few seconds, you will feel an intense heat in the tissues of the palms. Some very ancient cultures use this method preparatory to the laying-on of hands. A mode I find very useful incorporates creative imagery. Accepting the above-noted hand *chakras* as a basic assumption, use the imagination in every instance in which you reach for objects in the following manner. Look at your palms and note the depression in the middle of the palms, which forms a sort of well. Keeping your hands relaxed, notice what they feel like. In a normal state, you will feel nothing remarkable; however, this is what I want you to recognize first so that you have an idea of your own baseline feelings. Now, open your hand as wide as it will go, put your palmar muscles on stretch, and feel the increase in tone in these muscles. Relax your hand once more, and you will notice a tingling in the palmar surface of your hand. In the steps that follow, I would like to direct your attention to this sensation in a particular way.

THERAPEUTIC TOUCH SELF-KNOWLEDGE TEST #8: THE ENERGY CENTERS IN THE HANDS

1. Place your hands in front of you, palms up.
2. Test your hands for relaxation by moving them once or twice to make sure that the wrists are loose, almost limp.
3. Simply note what your hands feel like in this baseline condition. Do not touch them to each other; simply recognize what they feel like as hands.
4. Now, extend and separate your fingers and straighten out your hands fully—that is, put your palmar muscles on full stretch. Keep your hands in this position for the count of *15*.
5. Relax your hands and notice the tingling sensation of muscle tone in your hands.

6. Pay particular attention to the sensations arising from the wells of your palms. As you feel the tingling, see if you can sense as well a rhythmic pulsation arising from the well of your palm. The pulsation may also be accompanied by a sense of heat.
7. Once you have become aware of the pulsating sense of heat, I would like you to exercise this perception for the next three days by doing the following: In every act of reaching–from the act of reaching for your toothbrush when you first get up in the morning and thereafter throughout the day until you once again reach for your toothbrush before you go to sleep–reach out with your palm, instead of your fingers. During this act, feel as though you are reaching out with antennae that arise from the well of your palm. Know that "you don't stop at your skin" and see if you can pick up any change in sensation before you actually come into contact with the object you are reaching for. It is important to note that these changes will not announce themselves with the blaring of trumpets and the rolling of drums. They are subtle, and one must make oneself receptive to them. The bodily attitude one has is very much like what one has when listening intently, all senses quiet but acutely aware of change. This, as a matter of fact, is exactly the stance one has when doing the Assessment: It is a "listening" for change, and, just as when you listen intently for sound, you will find yourself not necessarily looking at the healee, but rather looking off in the distance, perhaps with your head cocked to one side, as you process the data coming from the healee's personal field via the energy centers of the hand.

If you give this exercise three days of honest effort, you will find a new universe of experience literally "at hand." One of the ways I enjoy these perceptions is to use this exercise to "listen" with my hands' energy centers to groups of flowers or plants by extending my hands near the groups of flowers or plants. I came across this experience quite by chance while trying to help an ailing *Aloe Vera* plant for a friend. Since then, I have enjoyed plants and flowers in a delightfully different way. Among the groups of flowers I have particularly enjoyed are the Columbine. It may seem like an odd preoccupation; but if half the world's population has been talking to plants with impunity, I can surely "listen" to mine!

6

"Unruffling" the Field

As we have seen, the Assessment is concerned with getting some data on the healee's personal field so that you can then intervene knowledgeably. This consists of sensitizing the hands in a way that makes it possible to become aware of the characteristics of that field through frequent experience and objective testings of oneself and then of learning from the experiences of those testings.

These characteristics of the healee's field were determined by noting differences as one symmetrically scanned the healee's field and noted any way in which the sensations felt in one hand of the healer deviated from the sensations felt in his or her other hand. The major sensations that healers have said they feel when doing this are feelings of heat, cold, tingling, pressure, electric shocks, or pulsations. All of these sensations are very similar to the characteristics of the field noted in the simulated games described in Chapter 3.

One of these sensations, that of the feeling of pressure, seems to be indicative of a kind of static condition in the field; perhaps the best description might be the word "congestion," as that word is used in the literature on acupuncture to indicate a blockage in the meridians through which the *chi,* or vital energy, flows through the body. It is said that illness is caused by this congestion, which can then be relieved by the stimulation provided by the appropriate twirling of needles in the acupoints of the affected meridians.

When one feels this sense of congestion during the Assessment of Therapeutic Touch, it feels as though there is no movement in the energy field in that particular area of the person. One gets a sense of a static state, and it feels very much like the pressure most people will feel when they are doing the exercise using the cotton (see Chapter 3). In the words of one of my students, the field feels "ruffled"—the pressure gives it the sense of having many densities. A biophysicist who took one of my workshops said that the reason for this feeling was that, as the hands moved over the affected areas of the field, they picked up positive ions. Positive ions are formed when an atom loses an electron for some reason. Although the effects of ionization on human physiology have been studied for over sixty years, the understanding of these effects is still in its infancy.[1] Positive ion loading has been noted in crowded and congested locations where feelings of lethargy, headache, irritability, and symptoms stemming from inflammations of the mucosal tissues have been noted to prevail. On the other hand, a prevalence of negative ions has been noted in areas in which people report feelings of well-being, such as sites near waterfalls and in mountainous terrain. At present, the most frequent use of negative ion concentrations is in therapy for extensive burns of the body.

It is difficult to describe the feeling one has in noting this pressure; the nearest description I can think of is that it feels similar to what a person with edema might feel on a hot day, a sense of fulness in the tissues that makes the skin feel drawn and tight. It is not a pleasant feeling;

[1] Joseph B. Davis, "Review of Scientific Information on the Effects of Ionized Air on Human Beings and Animals, *Jl. of Aerospace Medicine* 34:1 (1963) p. 1. N. Robinson and F.S. Dirnfeld, "The Ionized State of the Atmosphere as a Function of Meterological Elements and the Various Sources of Ions," *Intl. Jl. of Biometerology* 11:11 (1967) 279–288.

indeed, you will find yourself shaking your hands or wiping them to get rid of the feeling. These gestures seem to work, for once you do shake or wipe your hands, you can feel energy flow again—or, at least, you do not feel the pressure.

This simple experience gives one the rationale of what to do for the healee, and that is to move the area of that person's field where the congestion has been felt. You will find that if you place the hands with palms facing away from the body at the area where you felt the pressure and then move the hands away from the body in a sweeping gesture, the sense of pressure seems to be relieved in that space. I find it most useful to make the sweep downward, following the direction of the long bones of the extremities nearest the area of congestion or to make the sweep perpendicular to the body surface itself. I find that the sweep feels as though I were actually pushing a pressure front. The feeling of the energy flow that follows the sweep is more difficult to describe. The nearest analogue is the feeling one gets as the hand is placed under a tap of running water; it does not feel like the water itself, the energy feels like the bubbles in the water flow.

We have called this sweep of pressure areas "unruffling the field"—a strange name, but a very descriptive one, for after one has done this motion several times, the "ruffle" effect previously noted seems to be smoothed out. The freeing of this bound energy, however, will not last long; but it does give the healer access to a mobile field, and thus the subsequent transfer of energy, which we shall discuss in the next chapter, comes quite easily. The major purpose of this act, therefore, is to free this bound energy, to get it moving; and this freeing of energy seems to facilitate the healing act itself. After one finishes this phase of Therapeutic Touch, it seems useful—that is, it "feels better"—for the healer to shake, wipe, or wash the hands. I do not know why one feels so refreshed after doing this, however, it is a common practice among healers. I have found that if one adds about a teaspoon of coarse sea salt to the water, the hand washing is particularly stimulating.

I have found it very useful to "unruffle the field" in several specific instances. Used as one long, sweeping motion, it is very useful in the soothing of babies (see the story of Susan in Chapter 2). I've also found it useful in cases where there is pain, such as arthritis, edema, headache, burns, gastrointestinal upsets, or tension. In the latter case, when there is tension, it seems to be very useful to "unruffle" in the area behind the neck and shoulders of the healee, keeping the wrists loose but the motions purposeful.

As has been noted previously, there are no miracles in Therapeutic Touch. Although "unruffling the field" will sometimes relieve symptoms, more often, it seems that the act allows the healee's field to mobilize its own resources so that self-healing can occur. At best, it has to be acknowledged that there is really very little we truly understand about the dynamics of human field interaction, and so it is the better part of wisdom to experiment individually in this area and then build up a personal repertoire of therapies. If you do decide to experiment, however, I would like to share with you a precaution suggested by Ms. Kunz, which, I am sure, has been one of the major reasons why Therapeutic Touch has proved so safe both for healee and healer. This suggestion is to work very gently and for a very short space of time (no more than two to three minutes) on children, particularly if they are very young, on very old people, on very debilitated people, and in treating the head in persons of any age. I have written above about the "different" time that seems to be involved in Therapeutic Touch; frequently, much can be accomplished in what we would ordinarily consider a very short time. Secondly, one can always go back and treat the healee further, if it seems necessary. Precaution does have its places, and this is one of them. Give yourself an opportunity to test out these ideas on Therapeutic Touch, and then work from that base of experience as your own judgment dictates. We shall discuss this in more depth in Chapter 11.

7

Directing and Modulating the Transfer of Human Energy

As an open system, man is always engaged in the transfer of energy. In actuality, the physical make-up of his body is in constant flux—in essence, no more than a locus for a constant in-put, through-put, and out-put of human energies. One of the effects of this constant movement of streams of molecules through our bodies can be experienced by noting the body's radiation of heat. This through-put can be measured; it is based upon a random movement of energy. However, what we are attempting in Therapeutic Touch is the *specific* transfer of energy; we are engaged in a knowledgeable direction and modulation of those energies in a therapeutic manner.

It has often seemed to me that the expertise of the healer is in direct proportion to his or her ability to direct and modulate the transfer of his or her energies to bolster the deficit of energy of an ill person. Directing energy can be done in two ways: Primarily, energy is directed in a specific manner from the excess store of energies of the healthy person, the healer; and, in addition, the knowledgeable healer can direct energies from one place to another within the body of the healee. It should be said quite frankly that there is little to support that this actually occurs, for at this time there are no accepted means of measuring this transfer; and black on white numbers are, in fact, the measure of reality in our Western society. The same must be said about the modulating of energy, however much there may be subjective improvement, to say nothing of the amelioration and/or disappearance of symptoms. The modulation of energy is concerned with a tempering of one's energy outflow to meet the needs of a particular healee. The ability to modulate energy flow derives, I believe, from the intentionality of the person playing the role of healer; it is a fine skill that is based upon much practice.

The underlying basis of the whole act of energy transfer is the Assessment (see Chapter 5). When the Assessment was done, we accepted the fact that man is symmetrical; and we looked for energy responses that were different on one side of the body from those on the other side of the body and noted where these differences occurred.

In order to decide what we do with this stored information, we once again return to the literature of the world. In this literature, we find another consensus (the first consensus is the limited expressions used by all healers to describe what they feel in the ill person that gives them the knowledge that the person is sick–sensations of heat, cold, tingling, pressure, electric shocks, or pulsations). The consensus concerning why the person is ill is most frequently stated in terms of there being an imbalance of energies; some say that the ill person is in disharmony with the universe or with a God or gods; others say that there is a disequilibrium between the *yin* and the *yang* factors in the individual, and so on. My next step is simply to accept these statements as valid, both on the basis of general concurrence of opinion and because these same reasons have been stated by many people of authority who come from far-flung corners of the Earth. All such statements basically agree with acceptable ploys I would use in another context–that is, if I were attempting to do research within a Western scientific framework, in which case I would call them basic assumptions. Therefore, the rationale I recognize that I can use in the transfer of energy is to try to make both sides of the ill person's field "feel" the same, so that the field is symmetrical once again.

Using this as a basic rationale, I now turn my attention to transferring energies of the appropriate type to balance the healee's field. It is now that I see the importance of the Assessment, for it gives me two pieces of information that will provide important clues on how to rebalance the healee's field.

1. The Assessment tells me where the imbalances (the "differences") are.
2. The Assessment gives me a sense of the nature of these imbalances—that is, they are hot, cold, tingling; or they feel like electric shocks, pressure, or pulsations.

Using this rationale as a rule of thumb, I now follow the logic one step further: If I use the localizations of where the "differences" are to decide where the sites are to which I shall direct my energies as healer, then I now turn my attention to the quality of those cues as indications of some way of modulating that energy. In general, my rationalization tells me that if I felt heat during the Assessment, then I want to balance the area by "cooling" it. The qualities of the other cues are equally suggestive: If the area felt cool, it needs to be warmed; if the cue was a sense of pressure, the area needs to be mobilized; the tingling needs to be quieted, the pulsations moderated and made rhythmical, and the electric shocks dampened or "sedated."

How does one learn to do this? Essentially, it is an interior knowledge that is based on a feedback loop within oneself. Again, let us play some games to simulate aspects of the experience, and then we can have a common base for further discussion.

THERAPEUTIC TOUCH SELF-KNOWLEDGE TEST #9: THE DIRECTION OF ENERGY

Remember that "we do not stop at our skin." In this Test, you will learn to become aware of directing energy down your arm so that its arrival in your hand *chakra,* will become apparent to your partner. If you are doing this test in a group, then divide into teams of two persons; if you are not with a group, ask a friend to play the role of Receiver.

1. When you have a partner, decide between you who will play the role of Sender and who will be the Receiver.
2. Sit at a table in such a manner that each of you can easily outstretch your right hand towards the other as if you were going to shake hands; however, do not have the palms of your hands touch.
3. You will find that it will be quite natural for the Receiver to lay the back of the hand lightly on the table, while the Sender tips his or her hand over that of the Receiver's. Do not have the palms of the hands touch. Keep the wrists loose and the shoulders depressed to eliminate any tension.
4. The Receiver will do most of the talking and will also act as the judge of the Sender's ability to direct energy. The Receiver will give the Sender directions somewhat as follows:
    a. Since you had the experience before of proving to yourself that "you don't stop at your skin" (see Chapter 3), close your eyes for a moment and see if you can feel what the energy making up the space just beyond your right shoulder feels like. When you can feel that energy, let me know.
    b. Now that you feel that energy, try to bring it down from your shoulder to your elbow. When you do so, let me know.
    c. Now, bring that feeling of energy down your arm from your elbow to your wrist and let me know when you feel it there.
    d. Now I would like you to feel the energy just beyond your right shoulder again; and when you do so, I'd like you to bring that energy down your arm to your hand and feel the energy in the energy center in your hand.
    e. Once more, I'd like you to feel the energy just beyond your right shoulder. This time, I'd like you to bring the energy down your arm to your hand and then leap the gap be-

tween our hands and have the energy touch my hand energy center.

5. The Receiver now "listens" for a response in his hand. As noted previously, the feeling of energy flow is subtle, but it will be a discernible difference. It will not be an exotic difference, it will be only a slight difference; but you will be aware of a definite change during Moment #2—you will feel different than you did during Moment #1. Simply remember: "Do not expect it to be accompanied by the blaring of silver trumpets and the rolling of drums!" You will find it to be quite a natural phenomenon, resembling the feeling of bubbles in flowing water.
6. When the Receiver becomes aware of the energy flow, he should now change roles and become the Sender. Repeat the Test.

I developed this game about three years ago and have found it to be most useful as an exercise, as well as quite a lot of fun. Since then, I have developed some variations, which I shall explain below. The key to expertise in Therapeutic Touch is practice, so avail yourself of every opportunity to gain this experience.

In addition to directing energy, it is important to know how to modulate that energy flow in specific relation to the healee's state. It is not enough to channel energy to an ill person; as a matter of experience, it seems that one can actually do more harm than good by simply flooding a weakened person with energy. As one begins to get some depth of understanding of man as an energy system, it also becomes apparent that there may be situations in which you might wish to energize one facet of an ill person's field while calming or sedating another. The combinations can be as varied as man is complex.

I find that the easiest way for me to conceptualize a modulation of energy is in terms of color. There are several reasons for this, but the most basic is that the colors we perceive are actually different wavelengths of energy. All cultures appear to recognize this difference, and many assign specific qualities to colors in their mores and taboos. Surprisingly, there is some general agreement on these values; there seems to be greatest agreement that the color blue will sedate, that the color red will stimulate, and that yellow will energize. Within my experience, I agree with these connotations, particularly if they are colored light rather than colors of pigment. I would like to share that experience with you in two ways.

THERAPEUTIC TOUCH SELF-KNOWLEDGE TEST #10: EXPERIENCE COLOR AS MODULATION OF ENERGY

For the purposes of this Test, you will have to explore your city a bit and find a church, synagogue, or mosque with good quality stained glass windows.

1. Go to the place you select at a time when the sun is shining through a stained glass window.
2. Sit or stand so that the colored light from the stained glass window falls upon your body; the best place seems to be the face.
3. With your eyes either open or closed, pay attention to the "feeling" of the color shining on you—that is, experience any change in mood you have when you move your body into the light, note any physiological changes you experience when the light is shining on you, and so on.
4. When you feel you have fully experienced one color, move so that another colored light from the stained glass window falls on your face or body.
5. Note particularly any change in mood or any significant physiological change (change in pulsebeat, rhythm and/or depth of breathing, and so on) that may take place following the change of color.
6. Write down your experiences for later reference. If you are doing this Test with a partner or with a group of friends, discuss your experiences.

I have found that the most satisfactory experiences that I've had with this Test have occurred when I have used a stained glass depiction of The Mother of the World. Invariably I find that the blue of this archetypal lady has such pronounced qualities that I have no difficulty recalling it at will whenever I wish to. Like the other games we have played thus far, this one also carries with it a quality that is not difficult to retrieve in one's memory bank.

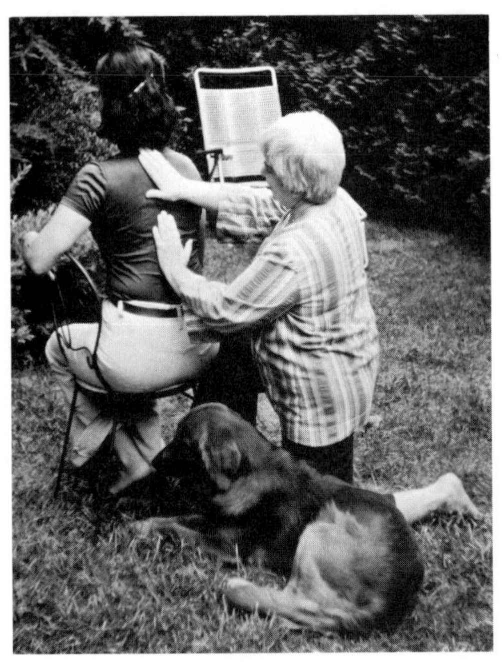

DK transferring energy from upper to lower hand on spinal column.

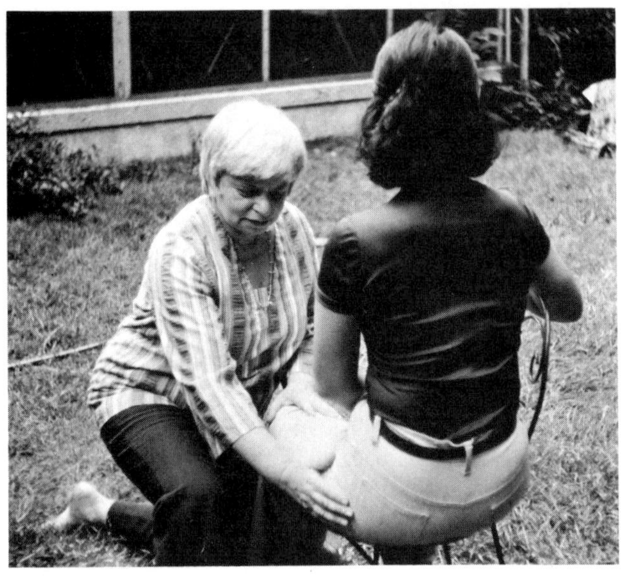

DK transferring energy from hip to knee.

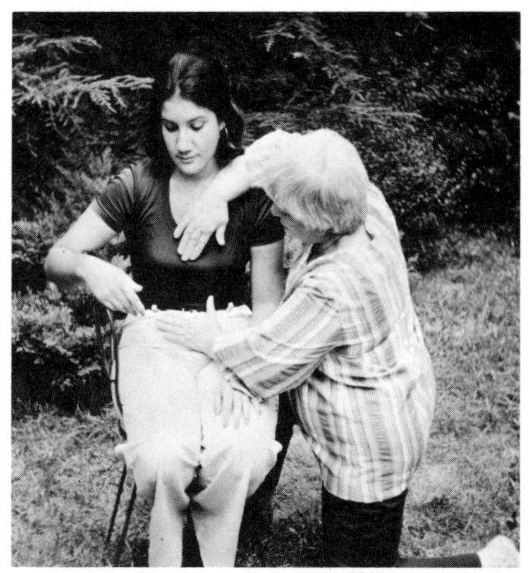

DK transferring energy over heart chakra to solar plexus chakra.

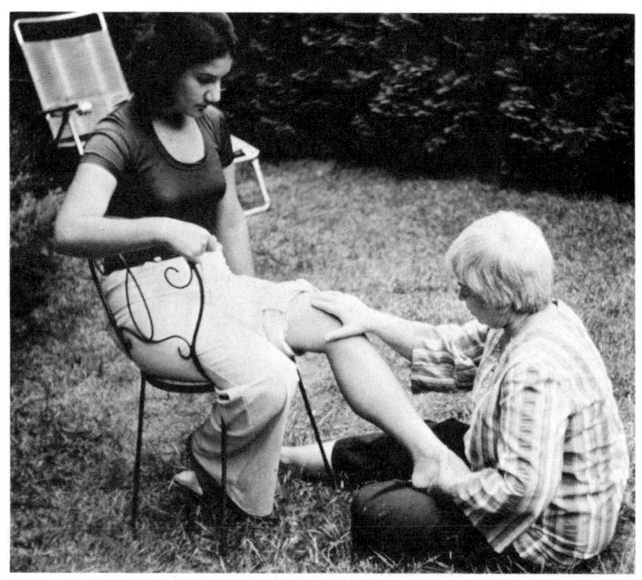

DK transferring knee chakra to foot chakra.

THERAPEUTIC TOUCH SELF-KNOWLEDGE TEST #11: THINK "BLUE"

Once one has had a conscious experience of color as energy, it is not difficult to recall, reminisce, or meditate on a particular color, a series of colors, or innumerable combinations or blendings of colors.

Although this Test can be done anywhere, a quiet spot is very helpful. Before you begin, give yourself a few moments to relax and change the pace of your previous preoccupation.

1. Close your eyes and choose a color you would enjoy experiencing again.
2. Visualize the color you decide upon. Satisfy yourself that it is the shade you want; however, if this makes you anxious, simply accept whatever shade comes to mind.
3. Try to get a sense of the color you are visualizing. Ask yourself: What is it that I experience when I think "blue?"
4. Note your impressions just as they come to mind and allow your mind to associate ideas. If you find your mind wandering, gently bring it back to the question: What is it that I experience when I think "blue?"
5. When you have experienced the color blue to your satisfaction, go on to another color. If necessary, and if you wish, this Test can be extended over several days. However, most people will find that a concentration of five minutes or, at the most, ten minutes, is adequate for later recall. Do not allow yourself to become rigid in your expectations. Experience all the dimensions of which you are capable when you ask yourself the question: What do I experience when I think "blue?"

THERAPEUTIC TOUCH SELF-KNOWLEDGE TEST #12: MODULATING ENERGY

Now that you are aware of how you react to color, we can put together some of these experiences in order to practice modulating energy.

1. This Test is based on *Therapeutic Touch Self-knowledge Test #9: The direction of energy* (see above). Choose a partner and sit opposite each other at a table or at any other object that will allow you both to rest your lower arms and hands in an outstretched position.
2. Decide between you who will be Receiver and who will be Sender.
3. The Receiver's hand can lie on the table so that the back of the hand lightly rests on its surface. The Sender's hand will be uppermost, arm relaxed on the surface of the table, hand overlying but not touching the Receiver's hand.
4. In this Test, the Receiver does not give directions; the Sender decides for him- or herself which of the three colors–red, blue, or yellow–she wishes to send.
5. After spending a moment to recall his or her experience with one of the colors–for the sake of an example, let us use the color red–the Sender tries to replicate within him- or herself the feeling tones he or she associates with that experience.
6. When the Sender feels he or she can both visualize the color red and recall the essence of the "feeling" of red, he or she tries to replicate that experience–that is, to actually re-experience the characteristics she felt when he or she had previously asked him- or herself: What do I experience when I think "red?"
7. Once he or she has recalled that experience of red, he or she simulates the associated feeling tone within him- or herself and directs that that feeling tone be concentrated at or near her right shoulder.
8. Bring those feeling tones associated with the color red fully to awareness and direct them, as in Test #9, down the arm towards the hand.
9. Direct those energies to leap the gap between your hand and that of your partner, and then experience them impinging on your partner's palm.
10. The trick of the game is for the Receiver not only to feel the impingement of the Sender's energies but to be able to interpret which of the three colors–red, yellow, or blue–the Sender transmitted.

11. Whether the Receiver guesses the color correctly or not, after he or she has had one chance to name the appropriate color, change roles and try the Test again. Both of you will be amazed at how quickly you can pick up this method of modulating energies. If, by chance, one of you is consistently not able to interpret the colors correctly, change partners with another couple.

Since I discovered this game, I've had lots of fun devising variations —for instance, instead of sending colors to your partner, try sending hot or cold. Learning in this manner can be fun, and, indeed, it should be. It is particularly interesting to play this game with perceptive children.

Once you have had some measure of success with these games, the rest of the techniques are simple—simply because they are so natural.

In physics, it is well known that it is the surrounding force field that carries the charge or electrons between objects, regardless of whether those objects touch—that is, come in contact with each other—or not.[1] This occurs because the outermost electrons of many atoms are bound very loosely and can therefore be easily dislodged. Something analogous to this seems to happen in Therapeutic Touch. When the person playing the role of healer turns his or her hands so that the palms face each other, what can be called a force field is evident between the hands; and it is this field that seems to carry the energy involved in Therapeutic Touch from the healer to the healee. The field I refer to is very similar to the one you built up in *Therapeutic Touch Self-knowledge Test #1: You do not stop at your hands.* As a matter of fact, some Krieger's Krazies center by practicing that hand game and then go on to place the field over the area to which they are going to do Therapeutic Touch. This is most comfortably done by placing one hand on one side of the healee's body and the other hand on the other side; however, it can also be done with the hands side by side or in any other suitable position. Once you are aware that a force field has been established, direct the energy down your arm to the person you are trying to help. In the same manner, you can modulate the energy as necessary. As in all of the games in this book, do not believe anything unless you feel assured that it is a reality. One of the ways I've checked myself in the past to test whether or not I was

[1] Paul G. Hewitt, *Conceptual Physics,* 3rd ed. (Boston: Little, Brown and Co., 1977), pp. 324-325.

feeling something different between my hands when I built up a field was to remove one hand and feel the space elsewhere for a while. If it again felt different when I resumed the field, then I was willing to say, "Yes, it is different!"

A final word is perhaps appropriate here, and that is to reiterate the importance of experience. Practice on your relatives, practice on your friends, and if you have neither, then practice on your animals or your plants. Please remember that without practice all of the words you have read thus far are merely an intellectual exercise.

8

The Personal Experience

Although the answer to the question of what it is that actually happens in the healing act is still poorly understood, it is important to acknowledge what has been experienced—what seems to be the case—as well as what is actually—that is, objectively—known. This personal attack at the frontiers of knowledge, has good support in the Western scientific frame of reference; it is called modeling and provides a base for the visualization of the processes that underlie the conceptualization and subsequent development of theory.

So far, we have discussed the more basic aspects of Therapeutic Touch. With experience, you will find that the techniques and their many variations will arise more from innate ability than as the result of a recipe. In regard to the latter, as I have mentioned above, one of the unexpected aspects of Therapeutic Touch is the way it uses time. Within the Therapeutic Touch reference, time is not linear. It would take another book to discuss this statement in the depth it deserves; at this time, let me simply say that there seem to be five distinct phases to Therapeutic Touch:

1. Centering oneself.
2. Making an assessment of the healee.
3. "Unruffling" the field.
4. The direction and modulation of energy.
5. Recognizing when it is time to stop. One stops when there are no longer any cues; that is, relative to the body's symmetry there are now no perceivable differences bilaterally, between one side of the field and the other as one scans the healee's field.

Nevertheless, these phases will not necessarily occur in that serial manner. I have touched on this above: You will find that, even as you approach the healee, the proximity of your energy field, the specificity of your attention, the innate relationship itself, and perhaps innumerable other factors which we do not as yet recognize, may begin to affect the healee in a therapeutic manner. In a similar manner, you will find that even as you are engaged in the "unruffling" of the field or the direction or modulation of energy, your assessment of the healee will sharpen considerably. You may also find that measurable physiological changes will occur in the healee in unexpected time frames.

Another interesting factor that one realizes with experience is that there are various states of consciousness to be experienced during Therapeutic Touch. For instance, I have noted that I have had experiences in five different modes or states of consciousness during the Assessment. The first mode has been discussed above (Chapter 5) in reference to the recognition of temperature differential. A second state occurs somewhat automatically and feels as though my hands were being drawn to a particular area somewhat as a piece of iron is drawn towards a magnet. The third case is really an analytical state of consciousness where I am saying to myself as I make an Assessment: Now I feel an imbalance in this person's symmetry here, here, and there. What can that information mean in terms of my previous experience and learning? A fourth state of consciousness is intuitional. It usually comes as a flash, and I simply know that I know.

The fifth state of consciousness is very difficult to verbalize. The nearest description I can come to is that there seems to be a deep level of one's being, beyond the superficial level of unconscious thoughts, where it is possible for one facet of an individual's personality to be in dialogue with another facet, and it is from that depth that the Assessment arises. There is a considerable depth to be explored experientially in the Therapeutic Touch process. One facet of such exploration concerns how the healer processes information. We will discuss various theoretical hypotheses in Chapter 9; for a moment, let us take a look at the question of information in-put from an experiential point of view.

A common experience of persons who use Therapeutic Touch consistently is a significant change in lifestyle. I ask my students in the Frontiers of Nursing course (the Krieger's Krazies) to keep a journal, and from over 300 of these graduate student journals, I find that, on the average, it takes about two to two and a half weeks of continued involvement in the use of Therapeutic Touch for a change in lifestyle to occur.

Most frequently the change is based on an increased use of natural faculties—faculties that our culture usually allows to lie dormant within us. One such faculty is that which we have called telepathy. This faculty does not announce itself dramatically; rather, it appears unobtrusively and touches one's life in small, frequently routine ways. Almost every person has had experiences, particularly when engaged in routine tasks—washing the dishes, mowing the lawn, and so on—when suddenly a thought arises about a particular person—let us call him "Joe." You think to yourself, "Gosh. I haven't seen Joe in a long time. I should phone him now." As in the classic story, you go to the phone to call Joe, but on the way the phone rings. You answer it, listen a moment and then say, "Hello Joe!" The person who called is the individual you were thinking about a moment ago. This is an act of synchronicity, of course, and we have all experienced them in one form or another. What is interesting about the person who is deeply into Therapeutic Touch is that these incidents occur frequently, frequently enough that one can test the situations often and thus get a very good idea of the reliability of this mode of communication. Once one understands the limitations of its reliability, this means of communication can be used just like any other tool.

Initially, it may come as a surprise that telepathy could be a by-product of Therapeutic Touch; however, upon reflection, it becomes clear how this can happen. My own rationale follows these lines: In my conception of the dynamics occuring during the Assessment, it seems to me that as the person playing the role of healer scans the healee and tries to make sense of the garnered information, in his or her mind he or she uses the healee—that is, his or her impressions of the healee—as a model. He or she then tries to replicate this model; that is, in his or her attempt to understand how he or she can best help the healee, he or she (perhaps unconsciously) tries to attune him- or herself to the differences which he or she becomes aware of as he or she scans the healee. In some such manner as this, he or she begins to understand the healee in relation to him- or herself. I think that in the healing act itself, during the directing and modulating of energy, exactly the opposite happens: In this case the healer uses him- or herself as the model, and, through a knowledgeable transfer of energy, he or she helps the healee to emulate his or her own healthy self.

To carry the occurrence of telepathy in persons deeply and consistently engaged in Therapeutic Touch to its final conclusion: It would appear logical, given all the assumptions that the above modeling implies, that if the healer is trying to get in to intimate touch with another, to learn to react sensitively to that person's "vibes," it should not come as a surprise that he or she is going to succeed in developing latent abilities in communication. As a highly personalized interaction, Therapeutic Touch provides a good milieu in which this can happen, and it does.

It is because the interaction between healer and healee can become so highly personalized that I call it a yoga of healing. Through it, one learns to develop many latent human abilities; as in yoga, the expert practice of Therapeutic Touch demands concentration and a deep sense of commitment to lifting a little the veil of suffering of living beings. It is an effort so constant that it can become a way of life.

During Therapeutic Touch, the person playing the role of healer literally becomes a human support system, supplementing the energies of the healee until the healee's own regenerative abilities can be mobilized in his or her own behalf. This dynamic human field interaction can reach very deeply within the psyche of both healer and healee. This will be discussed more fully in Chapters 9 and 10; at this time, I would simply like to bring it to the reader's attention.

Most illnesses invade the emotional domain as well as the physical; indeed, it is an accepted fact that between 50% and 70% of all illnesses are psychosomatic in origin. Therapeutic Touch can be very helpful in these cases once the person playing the role of healer has begun to understand her own emotions at an integrative level. In my experience, it seems that there is a direct relationship between the understanding the healer has of him- or herself and his or her ability to have a profound effect on the healee: the deeper the healer's understanding of self, the deeper the resonance with the healee's problems. I have found this of great help, particularly when doing Therapeutic Touch to people with frightening conditions, such as cancer, neurological problems, or psychiatric alienations. Knowledge of how to use one's emotions as a therapeutic tool can provide a means of "touching" people in ways that they may not ever have been touched before. Of the 4,000 or so people in the health professions to whom I have taught Therapeutic Touch, in workshops both in this country and abroad, many of the physicians and psychiatrists who take the workshop do so specifically for this reason—for it gives them access to their clients in a direct and thoroughly human manner. In order to help you get at this understanding and control of your emotions so that you can use them for therapeutic purposes, I would like to play some more games with you later in this chapter.

As noted earlier, Therapeutic Touch has been called a healing meditation by Peper (see Appendix II). I agree with that description, for the primary act in Therapeutic Touch is to center, and one of the most characteristic facets of its process is that the healer stays on center throughout the entirety of the Therapeutic Touch interaction. In actuality, it is from this center that the person playing the role of healer does his or her Assessment, directs and modulates energy, and maintains a posture of "listening."

During meditation, one feels as though one has stepped behind oneself, has become once removed, but nevertheless one maintains a full awareness of where one is and of where the healee is. With experience and a moderate amount of commitment to knowing, this ability can be developed so that the healer can learn to "look over his or her own shoulder" —that is, he or she can be aware, at any moment, even when interrupted, of where he or she is in the Therapeutic Touch process, of what the general state of the healee is, and of what he or she thinks he or she is accomplishing at that particular stage of Therapeutic Touch. These data are not simply based upon impressions but result from a consistent willingness on the part of the healer to test him- or herself against physical reality.

There is little place for wooliness of thought in Therapeutic Touch. Although our culture enjoys a good story, which encourages exaggerated use of adjectives and superlatives, this is a verbal luxury the healer cannot afford, at least in terms of her own interior dialogue—in the place where she evolves her self-image. At least in these private recesses of herself, the healer must accept only truthful and objective evaluations of what has transpired during his or her engagement in the Therapeutic Touch process. To overexaggerate carries the seed of fantasy and can lead to outright kookiness. You will find that, in actuality, objective testing of oneself strengthens one. There is so much in this form of healing that depends on "feelings"—which are, of course, subjective in nature—that it is critical to understand for oneself the clear signs of demarcation between imagination and reality. As is the case with the other experiences in Therapeutic Touch, once you understand your own frame of reference, even your imagination can be used as a therapeutic tool.

A game I would like to play with you now attempts to get at this kind of testing of oneself.

THERAPEUTIC TOUCH SELF-KNOWLEDGE TEST #13: THINK "LOVE"

This is a Test that you can do by yourself in any place that will allow you a few moments for quiet self-reflection.

1. Sit in a comfortable, posturally aligned position.
2. This Test is most easily done with the eyes closed; however, it is not entirely necessary.
3. Turn your attention inward and think of somebody you love, actually visualizing him or her.
4. While visualizing, send that person your love.
5. After sending loving thoughts to that person for several moments, continue the process but think to yourself: "What do I feel when I think 'love'?"

6. Fully experience your emotion; recognize and explore the "vibes" of it.
7. Try to articulate to yourself the tonal quality of this emotional experience; note any associated ideas that come naturally to mind during this time; note any other perceptions you may have. Do not force these associations; allow them to arise naturally, effortlessly, and spontaneously.
8. Now, turn your attention to the visualization of the person to whom you are sending thoughts of love, and try to imagine yourself standing beside that person.
9. Try to get a sense of the situation that person is in, particularly in reference to its emotional context.
10. Make note of your impressions of this context.
11. Gently bring yourself back to the situation you are actually in, open your eyes, and write down your impressions, noting the time and date of this experience.
12. At a mutually convenient time, but as soon as possible after this experience, communicate with the person you thought of and find out what the actual circumstances were at the time you did this Test. Be sure to get the information from that person first, and then share your experience with him or her if you wish.

There are innumerable variations on this game that one can play. The important part is to get back objective feedback from the individuals involved. If you can be impersonal when you are checking the real situation with the other party, then you can assure yourself of an objective evaluation of your impressions. In the context of this Test, it does not matter whether it turns out that you are right or wrong. What matters is that you know the quality of your own ability in an objective manner. It is on such a reality base that you can learn about *you*—a most important realization, if you want to play the role of healer.

Both the healer and the healee have experiences during the Therapeutic Touch process; however, it is of interest to note that they have different experiences. Perhaps this is most clearly demonstrated in a study reported by Peper and Ancoli on Krieger doing Therapeutic Touch on a group of four patients from an outpatient pain control center of a large hospital, a study which has since been replicated.[1] These show consistent electric encephalographic findings (see Appendix II). In each case, the patients went into a low amplitude alpha state, a state of calmness and well being from the onset of the Therapeutic Touch treatment and stayed there throughout the process. The patients were not aware of this; all they felt was that they were in a relaxed state of well-being, and they enjoyed the experience to the extent that they were all willing to volunteer for further studies on Therapeutic Touch. On the contrary, the person playing the role of healer went into a rhythmical, very high amplitude beta state (with all known extraneous artifacts controlled), which is indicative of a state of deep concentration similar to those occuring in mature meditators.

In addition to the symbolism the experience holds for both healer and healee, which we shall discuss in Chapter 9, the most significant reaction to Therapeutic Touch that the healee has is a rather pronounced relaxation response that has a characteristic pattern observable by others watching the process. The occurrence of this relaxation response has had a very high reliability over the past four years that I have noticed it; in fact, the reliability is so high (it will occur in about 90% of cases) that I use it as a test when skeptics challenge that "something" is happening in Therapeutic Touch. In these cases, I tell an objective observer, or the skeptic himself, the particular signs of the relaxation response I would expect to be observable on a particular healee (a role for which there are always volunteers in any audience) without the healee's or the audience's knowledge, and ask that observer simply to tell the audience what he sees after the healee has been treated by Therapeutic Touch. The signs which will occur are:

1. The voice level of the healee will go down several decibels.
2. The healee's respirations will slow down and deepen.
3. There will be some audible sign of relaxation in the healee, such as a sigh or a deep breath; or the healee may say something such as, "Oh, I feel so relaxed."
4. There will be an observable peripheral flush, a pinking of the skin, apparently due to a dilation of the peripheral vascular

[1] Erik Peper and Sonia Ancoli, "The Two Endpoints of an EEG Continuum of Meditation" (Paper presented at Biofeedback Society of America Conference, Orlando, Florida, March 1977).

system in the healee. This peripheral flush will be first noted in the face, but it is a general effect to the whole body.

It should be noted that these are observable data. The underlying dynamics have not been measured by sophisticated technologies within a controlled research design as of this writing; however, the clinical signs have held up after more than 100 repeated tests under the above-noted circumstances. I would suggest that the reader check out this claim for him- or herself once he or she has adequate experience. When it works, the preknowledge of this relaxation response is very effective!

There is another interesting aspect of the healee's experience, one that is relative to the question of the effect of persuasion, suggestion, the placebo effect, expectation, or faith. I do believe that they all play their parts in the healing process, and I know for a fact that suggestion in itself can be therapeutic. However, I have done two large-scale studies (130 subjects) and several small-scale studies that demonstrate no correlation of significance between professed faith that a healee will get well and the actual occurrence of healing in that person. These findings surprised me—as a matter of fact, that is why I repeated the large-scale study—but these findings have stood up even in the more informal studies. These results have led me to the conclusion that although expectation, suggestion, faith, and so on can effect the course of a person's illness, that effect lacks significance relative to a person's "cure rate," and this has been borne out by the clinical evidence.

Interestingly, the contrary has been true, and some of the best results of Therapeutic Touch have been on outright skeptics. In my experience, however, two personality variables—denial of illness and hostility—do have a negative effect on Therapeutic Touch, perhaps because they both may translate themselves graphically to the healer and inhibit the healer's efforts.

There is much about the experience of Therapeutic Touch that remains little understood or unknown. Therapeutic Touch reaches out to levels within us that have lain latent within our culture. Perhaps we have to learn to ask different questions of the universe than those we have articulated so far, and perhaps we have to learn to "listen" to the answers in new ways as well.

9

The Symbolic Experience

As can now be clearly seen, Therapeutic Touch is an experience in interiority. In this process, the major effect, if the opportunity is seized, can be an ever-increasing sphere of knowledge about oneself. The role of healer, with its many opportunities for direct confrontation with the frailities of the human condition, presents you with a rich lode of circumstances through which you can explore and grapple with the farther reaches of the psyche.

Focused by intentionality, guided by a motivation to help others attain a maximum state of well-being, and, most importantly, nurtured by a determination to understand why one wishes to help, the feedback from one's unconscious contents can become a life-long friend and teacher. In Jung's terms, it can become "an archetypal journey,"[1] a journey within to a place where the images and ideas we too frequently repress can provide the stuff for an astute modeling of our individual and personal relationship to the universe. Within such a modeling, the motifs, and therefore the meanings, of our interior experiences can become explicit and not just "reasonable" or "rational."

Finding that the psyche has a reality as "real" as that of the conscious, rational world, but that it must be understood within the context of the metaphor, may provide the open sesame to doors that have been little noticed in our age. Once we have learned not to fear the images that may arise from the representations we have stored in our collective unconscious, and once we allow ourselves adequate access to this secreted place, many linkages with our ancient and common heritage as Man can become discernible.

From this perspective, we can more easily perceive our common bond with others; and in this recognition, we may flash on why, indeed, we want to be healers.

These personal realizations do not usually fall into place easily in our culuture, for in our society stances of aggression rather than those of helping are the dominant and accepted mode. Nevertheless, where the stark contrasts of this time are depicted, in the playthings of our post-technological society—for example, in the movies, and in television and stage performances—we may see and recognize figures that are representative of our inner life. Frequently, this objective realization of our many connectivities to other beings may come into its fullness as the awkwardness of the novice who wishes to be healer are eventually worked through via experience.

The importance of helping the unconscious to emerge cannot be overemphasized. Whether as nurse, physician, therapist, or friend, helping or healing carries with it considerable responsibility, and under certain circumstances this may become a heavy load. The person playing the role of healer has need of a wealth of understanding coupled with a stable sanity. Just because you are involved in a nonorthodox lifestyle, people may seek you out in reference to nontraditional problems for which there may be no pat answers or even any precedents. Not always, but frequently enough, the core of the problem revolves around the *bêtes*

[1] C.G. Jung, *Four Archetypes,* trans. R.F.C. Hull (Princeton: Princeton University Press, 1969), p. 13.

noires, the beasts of the night, whom we unwittingly feed with the repressed contents of the unconscious, and in the weakened state brought about by illness they may prey upon the already anxious mind of the healee. If the person playing the role of healer has worked through insights into his or her own individual myth and from this understanding has evolved a strong philosophy of life, that person—without need of either philosophizing or psychologizing—can be very helpful as a model.

This, of course, can bring considerable problems in its train—problems that the reader should be aware of. As has been noted several times, Therapeutic Touch is a highly personalized interaction; and as such, there is ample opportunity for emotional involvements on the part of either or both parties. One can now begin to see why it is so very important that, from the beginning of his or her interest in healing, the person who wishes to play the role of healer understand his or her own underlying motivations. Given the personal nature of the therapeutic encounter, which may or may not use body contact, but which is practiced by the healer being in close proximity to the healee, almost every psychological ploy acted out during other personal therapies, such as psychotherapy, may also be acted out during the Therapeutic Touch interaction. At the least, one can become involved in occurrences of projection, identification, transference, and countertransference, and so the healer should be psychologically prepared for such encounters.

Projection may result in hostility, which, as noted above, can serve to nullify positive effects of the healing act. The caring, openness and nurturing of the healer can spark off the dynamics of identification in the healee, just as dependence and other passive qualities may stimulate the process of identification within the healer. Transference and countertransference commonly occur in everyday life and may intensify during therapeutic interactions. It is of interest to note Jung's findings that transference can lead to parapsychological phenomena.[2] Obviously, it is not the parapsychological phenomena themselves that one must be cautious of, but rather it is imperative to acknowledge the source of any paranormal happenings.

Because it is crucial to the understanding of self, I suggest that the reader who is seriously interested in pursuing Therapeutic Touch use every means to search out an understanding in depth of the fullness of

[2]C.G. Jung, *Memories, Dreams, Reflections.* Recorded and Edited by Aniela Jaffé. (New York: Random House, 1963), p. 137.

his or her personality. The symbolic is a very effective way of approaching the unknown within us, and so I suggest to my students that they learn of ways to draw out the images and ideas that lie dormant within themselves. There are several ways of doing this, but I find that the recording of dreams,[3] the drawing of mandalas,[4] and divination by means of consulting the *I Ching*[5] most useful. There are excellent books on the market in all of these areas. The few I recommend in the References can provide a base for the reader. In my experience I find that all three—dream content, the visualization of mandalas, and appropriate consultation of the *I Ching*—integrate the search for one's own authentic nature in a unitive manner which can be very creative as well as enlightening, particularly when a continuing record or journal is kept of the process. One such instance is the mandala illustrated in Figure 8. This mandala was drawn by one of my students, a nurse who worked in the operating room of a large hospital in New York City. The design in its entirety came to her "in a flash" as she was working and, during an operation, happened to look up at the lights over the operating table. The three brilliant yellow globes that dominate the mandala represent the triad of overhead lights above the operating table. A reflection of them forms the periphery of the central figure, which has a representation of the symbol for yin-yang at its center. The many dimensions of the experience are perhaps illustrated in the several circular rings, each segment of which is a different, though complementary, color. In the corners of the drawing are various symbols that are part of a symbolic translation of experience I invented which I call *Nursymbolese* and will describe more fully below. Finally, the entirety of the experience is encompassed within a strange geometric figure which is reminiscent of the Tibetan *yantra;* and, like the *yantra,* it serves to concentrate the attention on the contents of the mandala.

Symbolic content is also very powerful for the healee engaged in the Therapeutic Touch process. An experience of another nurse—I will call her Ann—illustrates this quite graphically.

Ann worked at night in the Recovery Room of a large Veterans Administration hospital and went to her classes at the university during the daytime. One night, she was doing some chores in the back rooms of

[3] Ann Faraday, *Dream Power* (New York: Coward, McCann and Geoghegan, 1972).

[4] Jose and Miriam Arguelles, *Mandala* (Berkeley: Shambala, 1972).

[5] John Blofeld, *I Ching,* The Book of Change (New York: E.P. Dutton & Co., 1968).

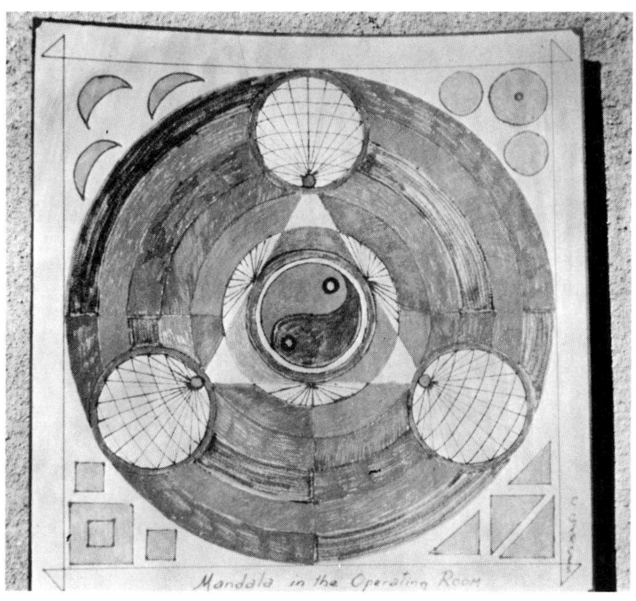

Figure 8. Mandala in the operating room.

the Recovery Room suite when she heard the sounds of a noisy disturbance coming from the forward part of the suite. She quickly came down the separating hall to find that a very large male patient who had undergone emergency chest surgery that evening was having a bizarre reaction to the effects of the anesthesia. The patient was thrashing violently in the bed, unconscious of the havoc being done to the equipment to which his body was attached and oblivious to the considerable danger he was causing himself. To prevent him from further harming himself, the charge nurse and a staff nurse were trying to restrain him.

Ann took in the situation at a glance as she entered the room, and she literally threw herself into the melee to add her weight as a restraining factor. To her surprise, she heard the charge nurse loudly say, "No! No! No! Do your thing! Do your thing!" Ann drew back, not quite understanding what the charge nurse wanted of her. The charge nurse continued, "Ann, do your thing! You go to that crazy class on Thursdays. Do your thing! Do your thing!"

Whenever I recall this story, I feel quite proud of Ann, for she did the right thing first: She took a moment to center herself, and then proceeded to do Therapeutic Touch. Much to her own astonishment and the delight of the other two nurses, within a few minutes the mindless violence of the patient stopped: He relaxed and fell asleep. He slept quietly throughout the remainder of the night, and at 8 A.M., Ann went back to her own apartment.

Curious as to what had happened, she returned to the hospital early. The patient had spent an uneventful day and by now was in his own room. Ann visited him there and questioned him casually about what he remembered of his experience the previous day. He remembered nothing. "However," he said, "I did have the wildest nightmare." "Would you care to tell me about it?" asked Ann. He would, and this is the story he told her:

> I dreamed that I was a lion in a jungle, and I was walking under the trees. In the jungle were three cannibals who lay hidden, and as I strode by they jumped on me. I fought mightily with them with all my strength because I knew that if I let up they were going to kill me.
>
> But they were too powerful for me and I felt my strength leave me. Just as I thought I would surely die, I looked up and there, as if in a cloud of green mist, I saw an angel. She smiled at me and I understood that if I could reach out and take her hand, I'd be safe.
>
> I closed my eyes and gathered my strength and then reached as high as I could. She put out her hand and helped me go into the green cloud.
>
> That's all I remember. The next thing I knew, I woke up, safe, and here in my own room.

This story of the green cloud is rich in symbolic content, but it is by no means unusual. Although we profess otherwise, we are still locked into a no-touch culture, and this is particularly and unfortunately true within the health field. However, the permission to touch is implicit in Therapeutic Touch, and from its enactment much formerly repressed material can well up in both healer and healee. As Jourard has pointed out, when a person touches another, he or she is in fact saying, "I want to share, I want to help"; and when the other allows his space to be penetrated and permits touch to occur, he is replying, "I want to share, I want to be helped."[6]

[6]Sidney M. Jourard, *Self-Disclosure* (New York: John Wiley and Sons, 1971), pp. 78–88, 146–150.

TABLE 9.1

GLOSSARY OF NURSYMBOLESE*

Symbol	Translation
△	Self
▽	Other (▽P patient, ▽N other nurse, ▽T therapist)
(group symbol)	Others acting as a group (e.g., cardiac team)
(dyad symbol)	Dyads (e.g., Mr. and Mrs.)
(dashed circle)	Localized human field
( )	Environmental field
(dashed circles around ▽)	Pregnancy
◇	Interaction in time (◇1 = 1st interaction, ◇2 = 2nd interaction, etc.)
(dashed diamond)	Open, nonmeaningful interaction
←→	Mutual, simultaneous interaction (MSI)
□	Formal (logical) analysis
(lower half-circle)	Other cognitive (unconscious or paraconscious) functions
(upper half-circle)	Decisive (conscious) act or realization
↑	Increasing complexity (growth, wellness; e.g., (▽ with ↑) = increasing complexity within other)
(complementarity symbol)	Complementarity
→, ←, ↗↙ (spiral, curved arrows)	Directions
⋘—	Past (e.g., (⋘ in box) = analysis of past history or deduction)
—⋙	Future

TABLE 9.1 (CONTINUED)

Symbol	Meaning
[symbol]	Moving at different rates of speed
FX/TIME	Function of time
[symbol]	A beginning (of a relationship)
[symbol]	Cyclic, repetitive action
[symbol]	Energy exchange
[symbol]	Flow of energy to or from self
+	Nursing (or healer's) observation
⊕	Nursing (or healer's) assessment
TT	Therapeutic Touch
☆	Peak experience
[symbol]	Low self-esteem
[symbol]	Low self-esteem of other
[symbol]	Confusion
[symbol]	Anxiety ([symbol] my anxiety [symbol] = his anxiety)
[symbol]	General (floating) anxiety
[symbol]	Depression
[symbol]	Pain
[symbol]	Ignorance (unsure, e.g., not understanding)
[symbol]	Indecision
⬡	End of process
[symbol]	End of transaction

*The individual reader is invited to devise personal symbols and add them to the Glossary.

If you would be engaged in Therapeutic Touch as a healer, you must accept the responsibility of acknowledging these implicit messages. As one way of doing this, I have devised a fairly painless method for bringing the content of unconscious acts of nursing into an individual's awareness, a method that I call "Nursymbolese." I would like to share it with you, since it is as applicable to daily life as it is to acts of nursing.

Nursymbolese is a kind of written sign language for translating daily personal as well as nursing acts into symbol. The *Glossary of Nursymbolese* (Table 9.1) is an open system that suggests certain symbols but also invites each individual to devise his or her own personal repertoire to correspond with that person's unique frame of reference. The symbols erase the sometimes frightening personal connotations that may be embedded in word and phrase, and the more indirect sense of meaning of the symbols may be accepted more willingly. At a later date, when the symbols instead of the emotion-laden words are analyzed, the unconscious content of the person's acts frequently arises to conscious awareness in a manner that may make them amenable to acceptance and integration into the self.

Nursymbolese can be used in several ways. As an example, one can imagine an incident of mutual and simultaneous interaction in which there was a decisive act: "He drew back as I approached with the hypodermic syringe in hand, and in that moment we both knew." This could be translated into Nursymbolese as follows:

Nursymbolese can also translate the flow of an act of nursing (or healing): "Jane rolled her wheelchair by me in the narrow hall. As I looked up from the medications cart, she caught my eye. I paused for a moment, and then, realizing that she was in a state of high anxiety, I went towards her."

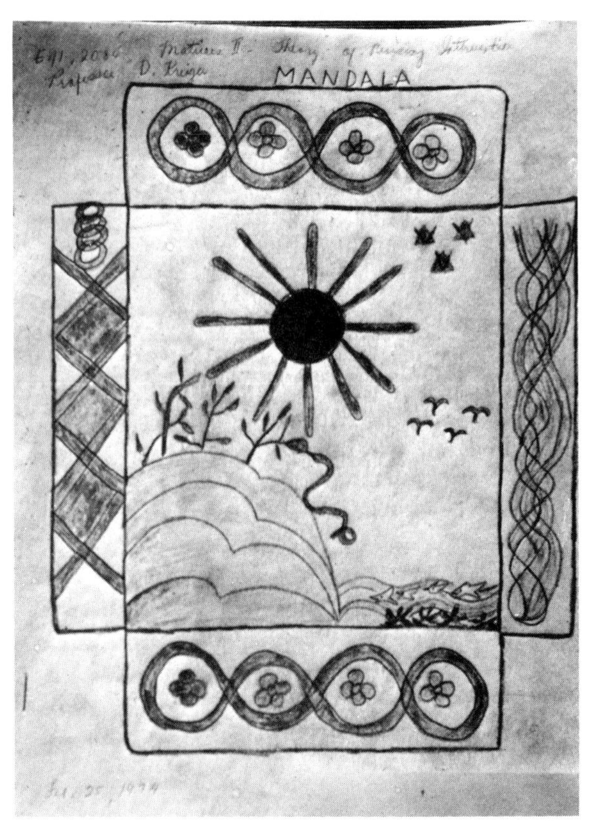

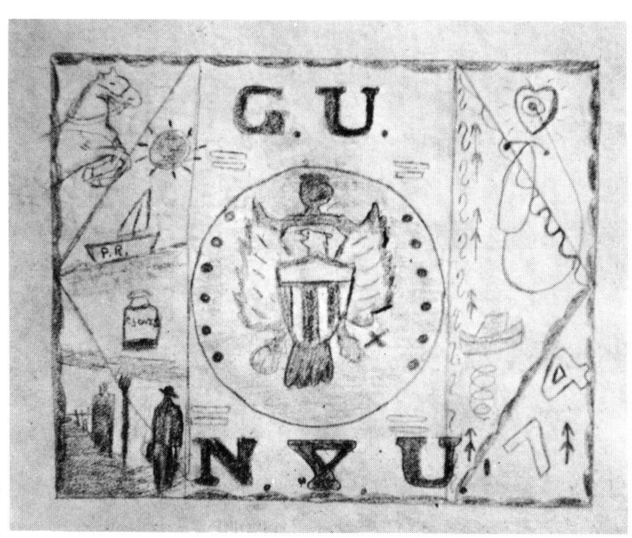

Mandalas by students.

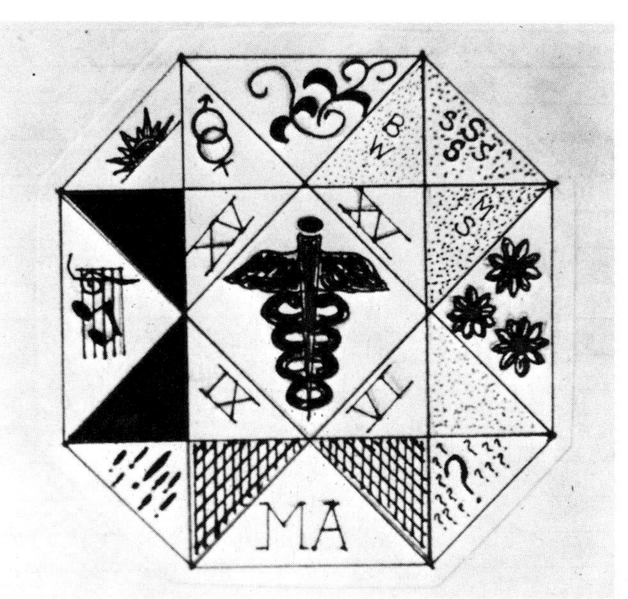

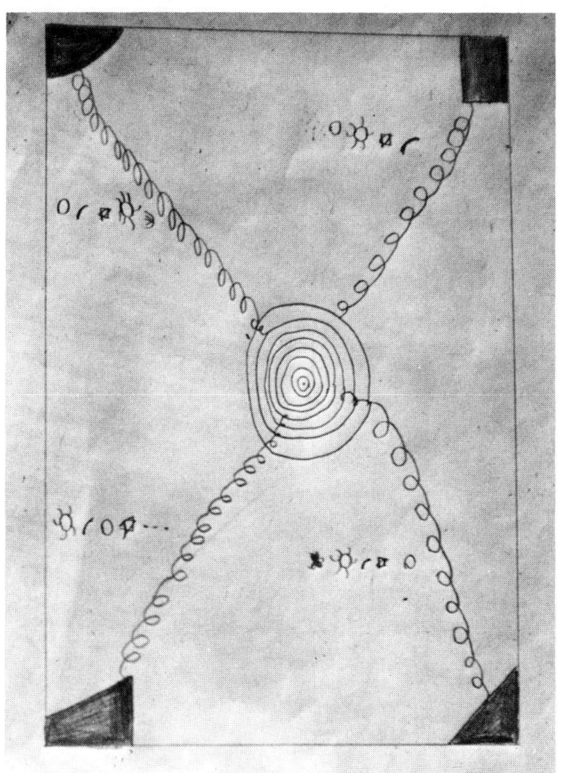

Mandalas by students.

As one analyzes the Nursymbolese, unconscious behaviors, cognitive bases for split-second decisions, and so on are brought to conscious awareness. Given this graphic understanding of one's own interactions, energy which may have been bound to action whose psychodynamic base may have been only dimly perceived is now freed to integrate into the depths of the self, and the healer is in a healthier position to understand and to help the healee. As awareness of one's unconscious involvement in daily acts of living deepens, one's personal symbolism unfolds gradually. As one becomes aware of the patterning of behaviors and recognizes that these patterns are meaningful, he or she is led towards a realization of personal wholeness, and it is this holistic point of view which can foster creativity. It is then that this person is, in Maslow's words, "most fully human."[7]

[7]A.H. Maslow, *The Farther Reaches of Human Nature* (New York: The Viking Press, 1972), pp. 55–101.

10

The Practical Experience

Therapeutic Touch has a high safety record for both healer and healee when it is done as suggested. It is obvious that if it is done otherwise, it is something else, not Therapeutic Touch. Nevertheless, it should be recognized that Therapeutic Touch is not a miracle cure, and sometimes it is not even a cure—but most times, it does help, and that can be invaluable.

To reiterate what has been said throughout this book, Therapeutic Touch effects a profound relaxation response; it helps to alleviate and, frequently, to eradicate pain; and, in a large majority of test cases, it does accelerate the healing process. Therapeutic Touch seems to work well with all stress-related illnesses; and, in my experience, it appears to have a significant effect on autonomic nervous system symptoms such as nausea, dyspnea, tachycardia, pallor due to peripheral vascular system contraction, and poor blood circulation in the extremities. There has been consistent clinical evidence that Therapeutic Touch increases peristalsis, and it can be used successfully with the colicky pains of unexpelled flatus and constipation. It has already been noted that Therapeutic Touch strongly supports the physiological development of premature babies and helps irritable babies to fall asleep—that last, at least, is worth a pat on the back!

This list could become very long and would serve little purpose; of more importance is the principle that seems to underlie the usefulness of Therapeutic Touch: It can be usefully used wherever there is an imbalance of energy. For instance, although at this writing I have spent about nine years doing research on the Therapeutic Touch process, I have no idea of its delimitations, of the illnesses with which it is always ineffective. The complexities of man are still little understood in our age, and there may be countless unknown factors that we may have no inkling of an idea about as yet but which, nevertheless, importantly affect healer and/or healee. On a purely pragmatic basis, Therapeutic Touch works, and therein lies its value. Research is sorely needed to make healing a more exact art, and Therapeutic Touch has been set up so as to include the most valid findings in its repertoire of techniques, but there are still too many questions left unanswered to develop a theory unencumbered by guesswork.

Clinically, there are many exciting indications that if we could ask the right questions, we could learn much about the human condition. In Chapter 2, I told the story of the young man in a wheelchair who was able to feel and describe the energetics of Therapeutic Touch even though his spinal cord had been transected and, neurologically, he should not have been able to feel anything.

To my personal knowledge, there are three other similar cases, so the experience does not seem to be happenstance. One instance occurred while I was on a trip to Alaska. In Anchorage, I gave a workshop on Therapeutic Touch, sponsored by both the Health, Education and Welfare Public Health Service and the University of Alaska, which was very well attended. As I went around to the various groups during the practicum, I came upon a young boy of eleven in a wheelchair, wearing a baseball hard-hat squarely on his head. We struck up a conversation, and he won me over completely when he said, "Well, I have leukemia (the hat was to cover the areas where his hair had fallen out as a result of chemotherapy), but don't worry. I'm learning biofeedback and I'm going to lick it!"

I asked him if he thought I might help him in some way, and he invited me to do Therapeutic Touch on him. As I scanned his field, I realized that the process had progressed quite far. I didn't think I could be very helpful in the short time we had together, and so I decided to see if I could help his paraplegia, which had disabled him considerably. I therefore started at the lumbar plexus, at the level of the hips. Within a moment after I set up a field, the boy began to describe to his father, who was by his side, feelings "like electric shocks" that were traveling through his pelvis and then down his legs. Right behind the sensations of electric shocks came feelings of deep warmth, which were also felt throughout the pelvis and then down both legs. As the warmth reached the lower legs and then warmed his feet, he burst into a grin from ear to ear and said, "Oh, Daddy! My toes are warm!" It turned out that that was the first time he had felt warmth or any other sensation in his feet in six months.

Another instance of a person feeling the process of Therapeutic Touch even though there was no neural circuitry to transmit the message occurred a few days after that while I was teaching class at New York University. I had taught the students in the Frontiers of Nursing class about the transference of energy, and they were practicing the exercise I describe in the Therapeutic Touch Self-knowledge Test #9 (Chapter 7). Out of the babble of voices that usually occurs when people find out for themselves that they can feel directed energy, there was suddenly a scream of surprise followed by, "I can feel it! I can really feel it!" It turned out that the person who called out had had irreparable median nerve damage when her hand had been cut in a car accident. She had previously had no feeling in that hand and, in fact, had cut her hand that morning while not paying attention to the position of the knife when slicing an orange.

I must say that the students were very good in testing her, for they first verified for themselves that she couldn't feel anything with that hand, and then they retested her while one of them transferred energy. Although the student felt nothing at all by contact, she clearly described her sensations of the transferred energy.

Two days later, I was in Boston addressing a large body of professional people in the health field. As an example of the wealth of unanswered questions we must accept the responsibility to explore, I cited the above-noted instances of sensation occurring in cases where we have heretofore believed it to be impossible. A young man in the audience challenged me to repeat that experience on him; he had also had severe median nerve damage and had lost sensation at the affected site. I did Therapeutic Touch to his hand, and he did experience the above-mentioned sensations to his full satisfaction, which he later willingly reported.

Another intriguing aspect of Therapeutic Touch is the question of time. One of the facets of this question concerns the rapidity with which measurable physiological factors are affected. For instance, there are a number of factors that can affect one of the components of the red blood cells called hemoglobin. However, during Therapeutic Touch there is a significant alteration of hemoglobin values even when all the known factors are controlled within a tight research design. I have witnessed hemoglobin changes of over 1.5 grams, which is an unusually large change, occur within as little as two hours after treatment by Therapeutic Touch, an exceptionally short period of time.[1] In four of the best controlled cases within this category, the blood system itself was out of order: One young man, twenty-two years old, had a terminal malignancy, two middle-aged women had pernicious anemia, and a third lady, about forty years of age, had an iron deficiency anemia. The young man's hemoglobin values changed within two hours. I was not able to retest the ladies' hemoglobin values until six days later, but at that time they all had significant changes in their hemoglobin although nothing was added to their treatment other than Therapeutic Touch.

Another curious fact about Therapeutic Touch is its relationship to certain materials, such as cotton. Cotton seems to act as a facilitator of healing. I found out about this in a rather strange way.

Some years ago, several persons and myself volunteered to close a camp we had been staying at, for it was Labor Day and the rest of the people wanted to avoid the holiday traffic. Those of us who remained worked as a group all morning and then broke up in the afternoon to finish up individual tasks.

Late that afternoon, I was working near the main house when I happened to notice one of the fellows, Bill, running down a path. He seemed to be in trouble, and I hailed him. Bill told me that his wife, Joan, was at their cabin and seemed ill, and that he was going to the main house to get a thermometer to check her temperature. I asked if he wanted my help; he said he did, and so I went with him.

Joan, who had seemed in excellent health that morning, looked very ill. Her temperature was 101.4°F, and she seemed very weak. We

[1] Arthur C. Guyton, *Textbook of Medical Physiology* (Philadelphia: W.B. Saunders Co., 1961), pp. 150–151.

took her down to the main house, and I did all the things I knew to bring the temperature down—aspirin, fluids, alcohol sponges (which I started by using washcloths to bathe Joan but changed over to the use of towels and to putting ice cubes in the alcohol bath because her temperature continued to rise).

At one point—when her temperature was 103° and repeated phone calls had not found any of the local doctors—I called the hospital to get permission to bring her to the Emergency Room. They told me to keep her at home, that they were in the midst of the largest number of accident cases in their history, and that it would probably be hours until they could get to her. Since I was a nurse, they felt she would be better off with me. "Keep her in bed and give her some aspirin," they said. "She'll probably be alright in the morning."

By evening, Joan seemed to be occasionally slipping into delirium. Her temperature had not gone down in spite of the alcohol baths, aspirin, and whatever fluids we could get in to her; and the possibility of encephalitis, which had occurred several miles away, entered my mind. About 10 P.M., we ran out of ice cubes; and Bill, who had been helping me with the alcohol baths, and I rested for a few minutes while one of the fellows went to a nearby bar to buy some more ice cubes.

I realized how ineffective our treatment had been and said to Bill, "I really don't know anything else to do, Bill. Would you mind if I tried Therapeutic Touch on Joan?" He gave me a startled look and said, "Mind? Look, Dee, I want Joan well. Try anything you think will help."

To give myself a few moments to decide exactly what I would do, I picked up the wet towels and took them downstairs. On the way back to Joan's room, I passed the first aid closet. The doors were partially open, and through them I could see a roll of absorbent cotton. Remembering that Mr. Estebany used to "magnetize" cotton for his patients, I picked it up and took it with me, even though I didn't know what to do with it. Returning to the bed, I had to kneel down because the bed was so low. I tried to recall by visualization what I had seen Mr. Estebany do with the cotton he prepared for his patients. Finally, I decided to separate a large piece of the cotton and put it over Joan's abdomen. I then placed my hands over the cotton and did Therapeutic Touch.

There is a discernible point in the Therapeutic Touch process when you know that healing is occurring. Just as I became aware of the culmination of that experience, there was an inexplicable incident: Out of a sky that had seemingly been cloudless, there flashed a huge jagged bolt of lightning, followed by a roar of thunder that shook the house. I had been deeply concentrating on the Therapeutic Touch process when this happened, and my reaction to this is not easily explained. Continuing the Therapeutic Touch process, I looked up and said quite calmly, "O.K., O.K. I know you want to help." Realizing what I had said, I looked at Bill, our eyes met, and we both roared with laughter. As the laughter subsided, still with my hands on Joan, I realized that her skin temperature had changed. I called to Bill on the other side of the bed to touch Joan's skin and let me know what he felt. "She feels cool!" he said, "Her skin feels cool!"

As we were discussing this, Joan began to stir and said all the classic things: "Where am I? What happened?" I asked her how she felt, to which she replied: "Feel? Why I feel fine." I asked her if there was anything she might like. Without a flicker of an eyelash she answered, "Well, yes. I feel hungry."

After some food, Joan fell asleep and slept soundly throughout the night. By the next morning, she felt well enough to make lunch for all of us, after which she and Bill drove back to Boston. There has never been a recurrence of this episode. I have, of course, thought about this strange happening from time to time. Joan is much too straightforward a person to have indulged in a put-on, and Bill is an analytical physicist, and the other people were verifiably stone sober.

I really do not know why the synchronicity of circumstances coupled the lightning and thunder with Joan's dramatic recovery. However, since that time, I've done considerable experimentation with absorbent cotton, and, as I stated above, I am convinced by experience that the cotton does act to facilitate the healing process.

I have used the cotton many times since, preparing it in exactly the same way I suggested to you in *Therapeutic Touch Self-knowledge Test #3: Intensifying the field effects* (see Chapter 3), and I find that it is especially good for musculoskeletal injuries. Over the years, it has come into use, particularly on surgical floors and in emergency rooms, when dressings are done, since the prepared dressing has a cotton filler. Since the hand does not have to come in contact with the dressing, sterility is maintained. I have also taught the technique to many athletes, who then do it to their own cotton and keep it in their lockers should they need it for future use. In the case of bicycle racers, marathon runners, and skiers, they keep it on their persons or among their equipment. Again, I do not know why it works, but it does; and to date, there have not been any reported untoward incidences to mar its record of safety.

11

You Can Help, You Can Heal

My major motivation in writing this book in this way has been guided by the persistent impression during nine years of postdoctoral research on healing that the therapeutic use of hands is a natural potential in Man which can be actualized under the appropriate conditions. My overriding feeling has been that if human beings can help each other in this most humane way, they should do so.

In most of the cultures of the world, healing has been surrounded by an aura of mystique, awe, superstition, and suspicion. My experience has demonstrated that there is no rational base for these negative emotions to bar any individual who has the intentionality to heal, the motivation to help others, and the willingness and ability to self-examine his or her desire to be a healer. The delimitations of one's ability to do this, I feel, are largely in the hands of each individual, literally as well as figuratively.

In order to bring out the nature of Therapeutic Touch clearly, so that you can decide for yourself whether you want to make it a part of your lifestyle, I would like to bring to your attention other research findings as well as several excerpts from the journals of persons who come from a wide spectrum of experience and who have chosen to try out the effects of Therapeutic Touch for themselves. The persons involved have given their permission for the publication of these experiential reports in the interest of furthering the understanding of Therapeutic Touch as a natural process through continued research, and so we are privileged to look over their shoulders, so to speak.

In Appendix I, you will find a form—Experiential Criteria During Therapeutic Touch—that I have developed to clarify what it is that happens to the individual who plays the role of healer during the Therapeutic Touch process. It has proved useful both in eliciting personal experience and as a tool to help summarize the Therapeutic Touch experience for oneself. For either or both of these reasons, I urge you to fill in the form for your own information, once you have some experience under your belt.

All of the questions relate to the individual's experiences during the healing act of Therapeutic Touch. The statements below represent only a sample of about 250 people in the United States and Canada who are engaged in the practice of Therapeutic Touch. The statements have not been altered in any way; however, they have been placed in the series by an impartial judge, who has been practicing Therapeutic Touch for several years, with what she judged to be an increasing maturity of experience. Below are several statements written in answer to the first question:

1. *How do you sense the external environment—that is, is there any significant difference in the manner in which you perceive things and/or people about you while you are engaged in the Therapeutic Touch process?*

◇ At this point (very early in my experience with Therapeutic Touch), I am unfortunately too aware of (that is, distracted by) the environment. The (heat of the) sun and cool breezes confuse me during the Assessment.

◇ At this point, as a beginner, I am not sure that I can really differentiate among the many things I have felt; but it seems that after centering, it is possible to concentrate more ably. Nevertheless, I think I felt more aware of the healee and less aware of the other activity about.

◇ The external environment is very important, but in my case I feel I have not changed in perceiving things and people, although the Therapeutic Touch process gives me a better chance to concentrate and center.

◇ The external environment and I become united at a deep level and interface with one another.

◇ No gross change noted. I'm really not paying attention. Lots of talking in the vicinity may be distracting, however, causing me to momentarily lose my center—I must work a bit harder to stay centered.

◇ It seems that I no longer pay attention to the external environment. Concentrating on what I am trying to feel, focusing attention on my hands—the rest seems to recede.

◇ I perceive beyond myself and the client, but it is with greatly reduced intensity. I see things around me—happenings—but I don't attend to them, like when I do TM (transcendental meditation). Some of the time my eyes are closed. Sounds are there, but I seem dissociated from them.

◇ The environment moves into the background (that is, the *specific* things in it), but the sense of its source or totality becomes strongly present. People are much more *real* to me during TT, that is, I sense their field or "being" and openness and feel an impersonal love for them, regardless of whether or not I "liked" them before.

◇ As my focus changes, external events fade, although I'm still aware of what is going on. My mind seems to split, so that one part remains in touch with events; but that becomes secondary to my other concentration.

◇ The environment is more beautiful and the people around me are, too.

◊ I feel more loving and accepting.

◊ Quiet, even though there are people talking. Peaceful.

One of the recurring themes that is of interest is the agreement that the healer engages in a highly concentrated act when doing Therapeutic Touch. Peper has called Therapeutic Touch "a healing meditation" in which the healer engages in a focused, passive act of intention. This intentionality is evidenced by "a preponderence of fast synchronous electroencephalographic activity" in a controlled study done during the practice of Therapeutic Touch (see Appendix II) which has since been replicated.

The second question asked:

2. *Do you feel any significant changes in your heart rate or respiratory rate or in your body's muscle tone or sense of energy flow?*

◊ No.

◊ I am aware of breathing deeper and of energy coming through me.

◊ Everything is slow, steady, smooth, and alert.

◊ When I tried too hard to make the energy flow, I experienced an increased pulse rate, flushing of the face, tightness around my neck and shoulder muscles, tingling in my fingertips, and an overall shakiness and weakness. When I stopped trying and just allowed the energy to flow, my breathing quieted and I experienced a sense of peace without the previous symptoms.

◊ Heart and respirations became slower. Shakiness or jitteriness disappeared.

◊ I haven't noticed any physiological changes such as variations in heart or respiratory rate, but my muscles seemed more relaxed, and I could feel the flow of energy at least part of the time. Thinking back now, I believe I noted that my respirations were slower and deeper.

◊ I feel more intense—as if all senses were sharper, although I am not using any particular one of the five "ordinary" senses. I believe there is an increase in my respiratory rate.

◊ Trying to maintain a centered place, I find I must stay relaxed—breathing slower and deeper. Don't notice heart rate or muscles that much. Can feel heat and prickling coming from my hands.

◊ I feel relaxed, focused, or centered and can feel an energy flow. I need to do Therapeutic Touch more to note other physiological changes.

◊ Not consistent, although if anything, I think respiration becomes slower and more regular. I've noticed that it works better when I'm relaxed—muscle tension or an uncomfortable position is distracting. Energy slows—I feel this in my hands—the palms and fingers—usually as a "prickle."

◊ I feel my muscles relax. I've never measured my heart rate before and after, but I feel that my rate increases. I never feel tired after Therapeutic Touch; at the same time, I don't think I've increased my energy level either.

◊ Yes. Respirations seemed to speed up at the beginning and then slow. When I was a healee, the energy flow during the peripheral flushing was tremendous. I felt very warm over the upper extremities for ten to fifteen minutes. It felt good.

◊ Muscle tone—I feel relaxed. The "parts" of me not directly involved (my legs) feel "dead," heavy, nonexistent. I cannot feel energy coming in, but I can feel the transfer of energy from the front of me and my arms—and I *know* it is flowing because I never felt drained. My hands get hot.

◊ Respirations become deeper and slower, the body becomes relaxed, and the hands get very warm as energy flows, even when I am "cooling" someone.

◊ No change in heart or respiration. If I seem to be a good channel, I notice that my muscles are relaxed. In fact, I probably use that as a sign that I'm doing well. I am sometimes aware of energy flow.

◊ Very aware of change in respiratory rate, which becomes lower, and energy flow, which feels centered and flows so that sometimes I really feel its circulation. An "inner voice" speaks when or if a connection with the healee is made. I am learning to listen better as that (inner voice) is the "me" that knows.

◊ My solar plexus feels more secure.

◊ Duration of my sleeping reduces to five hours from eight hours. I wake up spontaneously, fresh and relaxed.

◊ Very calm heartbeat and respirations. My muscles are very relaxed; I get a lovely sense of stillness and balance in the body/emotions/mind. Both energized and calmed at same time, as though I were in the midst of a space of stillness.

There seems to be general agreement in the answers to this question that when effort is "effortless," a relaxed focusing occurs. Although this seems a paradox, experientially it is not. One begins to recognize that the degree of awareness in TT (Therapeutic Touch) is not a function of exercising the "muscles of the brain" but rather that communication between healer and healee arises from the deeper realms of self, and that that inner space of quietude is a satisfying and enjoyable experience.

Below are the responses to the next question:

3. *In what way would you describe how you get meaning from your experience—that is, are you able to recapture the internal dialogue that goes on inside of you when you try to explain to yourself what it is your senses are telling you?*

◊ Not really.

◊ Not yet. I will need more time and experience to be able to answer this responsibly.

◊ I am not sure I understand this question, probably because I don't think I've been aware of the interaction between my internal dialogue and my other senses. The heat or tingling in my hands lets me know that something is happening.

◊ "Is this real—is this imagination?"

◊ I have a hard time convincing myself that I can actually feel much or that I can allow my impressions validity. In my mind, I tell myself to relax and take whatever comes, that the healing will happen, if it's meant to.

◊ I find myself looking for the meaning or the connection in the images that come into my view immediately after each image appears. That is when I stop the movie, think about the image, memorize it, and then allow myself to become recentered and restart the flow of images.

◇ I don't think there *is* an internal dialogue. *I* would cease to exist in that event. I am like an antenna.

◇ If the event touches my heart, then it has meaning, or it places me in a position to learn things.

◇ When I am fully participating, there is no internal dialogue.

◇ Sometimes I try to explain to myself what I am perceiving, and at those times, I don't feel that I accomplish anything. Nevertheless, I very definitely have an "internal dialogue" telling myself to pay special attention to what I am immediately feeling.

◇ I concentrate on any changes that might be occurring which I can perceive with my hands; then I try to determine if what I am doing is the best I know how to do in relation to the cues I am getting through my hands.

◇ At this point, I can only write that the dialogue is different from the usual, rational, step-by-step process. It seems rather like a knowing all at once—it's an all-or-nothing dialogue. It's much faster than the first process described.

◇ This is very difficult for me, because there are usually so many things going on in my head that it is difficult to stop it all and tune in to just one thing. I've found that if I just relax and let my mind be receptive, it works better. Also, I've found that at times I was looking for something else and wasn't aware that I was feeling in a different way even though I was not clearly visualizing the interaction with the healee in my mind.

◇ Since I am getting better at noticing differences, I'm also better at the subtler differences—for example, noticing "pulling" sensations, areas of "nothing" (which I'm beginning to correlate with energy deficits/blocks). Large areas of hot/cold differences I'm beginning to interpret as tension/pain, and side to side differences as "need differentials"—that is, when one side compensates for the other.

◇ I just try to tuck information away. I don't usually listen to internal dialogue. I am much more creative when I trust intuition and allow energy to flow quietly without giving expression to the reasons "why." I only feel confusion when I try to explain my feelings; my head often gets in the way. I know experience will bring a better blending here.

◇ It is little dialogue. It's more like listening alertly and intently but relaxedly to something that you trust instantly *without* the usual processes and steps of arguing clearly. I think of it as the *whole* guiding my own localized, focused intelligence.

◇ With me, it is almost a dialogue between head and hands, as if I try to remind my hands what they may perceive or as if I quickly interrogate them (in order to define and better remember) when they *do* perceive something.

◇ I think I'm trying to quiet the dialogue in my head. Sometimes I've had trouble with that, and my head has been saying, "That's probably not what you are getting from the other person but just your *own* sensations emanating from you." I need to keep my head out of it and just feel what I feel. I really believe my head (left brain, maybe!) just gets in the way. Later, maybe, I can listen to the dialogue in my head without having it interfere.

These answers indicate something of the difficulty one has in looking over one's own shoulder during TT. Once the healer has gotten beyond the stage of saying to him- or herself, "Now I do this and now I do that," he or she realizes that TT is an holistic engagement involving levels of consciousness which we are not usually aware of in our post-technological culture.

The next question deals with an area of ourselves with which we are somewhat more familiar:

4. *Have you noticed any significant changes in your emotions?*

◇ No gross change in reaction pattern.

◇ So far, I usually do not react, but sometimes I feel unsure about what I am doing.

◇ I feel more aware of emotions. I don't ignore them as I once did.

◊ I'm overreacting at times because I am seeing and feeling things that are exciting and that open up a new world to me. Previously, I believed that there was much "hocus-pocus" or possibly mass hysteria to explain away many so-called cures, miracles, and so on. I am much less apt to overreact now. Instead, I'm mindful of the energy field, of how I can protect myself and help others.

◊ I react much more calmly; I'm more centered. My emotions need not be involved in every interaction. They are uninvolved in healing, I think.

◊ Well, so far, the emotion I feel most is an insecurity and uncertainty about what I am trying to do; however, it seems that with practice, especially in centering, one's emotional response comes from a source of truth rather than just reaction.

◊ I feel calmer. If I am ineffective during Therapeutic Touch, a part of me feels panicky that I am unable to send or receive correctly; nevertheless, there is a steady, calm assurance that pervades in the background of my mind.

◊ I tend to overreact at times. I'm trying to control those emotions because I do not benefit so well from the experience.

◊ I consciously try not to react. Now, I have an entirely different way than usual of responding. It's not an intellectual or an emotional response (and difficult to describe). In healing, the energy comes from a different level, an intuitive source without value judgment, a completely honest place.

◊ I don't think I'm feeling very emotional *during* the process. I'm just focusing all of my attention to the person and the process. Maybe it will be different after more practice. Oh, I do feel calm. It's a really different way from the ways in which I usually react.

◊ Peace, well-being, a great impersonal love, a sense of warmth and glow in the heart *chakra* at times (as in fusion during group meditation). Unlike in the non-TT state during my day-to-day interactions with people; then I react *just right:* not too much nor too little. I only do what the accepted proprieties of conduct demand.

◊ I am feeling in a much more intense way. As when you asked about our feeling from the tree, I had tears. I have always had strong feelings from the redwoods—a sense of calmness, peace and strength —but today I was really aware of the feeling.

◇ I don't find myself reacting *during* the healing, but before. If I don't like the person—that is, if for some reason I don't feel "in tune"—I can't get focused. Also, if I am working with another healer with whom I do not feel in tune, I find it disturbing even to try to heal.

◇ My emotions seem quiet. I feel detached but have purpose. There is an intensity, but it is detached intensity. It almost seems that I am not trying, yet I know what I am doing.

◇ React in an entirely different way. I become more calm, "mellow" in feeling. Different from any other emotional experience.

◇ I am more calm, more receptive, more trusting.

◇ I have a sense of compassionate detachment.

◇ More aware of my inner being. More in touch with something I am not usually in touch with.

◇ Sensitivity and empathy increase along with compassion. I don't think I really feel I act differently, I just focus more intentionally.

◇ More and more I learn to be compassionate and detached at the time.

◇ Difficult to explain—but just as I feel an outpouring of energy, so, too, is there a giving or outward flow of love.

The next question asks:

5. *In what way do you use your memory—for instance, are you aware of a continuity of experience?*

◇ I can't remember.

◇ Yes.

◇ Because of my lack of experience, I would say that memory has not been put into play much yet. My memory isn't used too effectively—it seems that my excitement blocks recall processing.

◊ I talk to myself.

◊ The images that come forth are flashes, like an old silent movie. In order to remember an image, it feels like I stop the reel, memorize the image, and then continue to view the rest.

◊ I sometimes find it difficult to forget the previous patient when I heal the second one.

◊ Experience is obviously the basis of all correlations, so memory has served to provide some basis for validation as well as discovery. I am beginning to "sort" out some earlier experiences in terms of the present. During assessment, this comes to the fore.

◊ I do seem to enter a same state of mind each time I undertake Therapeutic Touch. It's similar to but yet deeper than, the state I find myself in when I'm examining my patients at the hospital—I'm tuning in to their story.

◊ I don't like to engage memory at all, if I can help it. Just be here, now.

◊ I make note of any temperature changes I feel so that I can go back to those areas after the initial Assessment. In the Assessment I make a mental note of where I notice differences. I keep this in mind during healing.

◊ I do have a continuity of experience. I like to write down my feelings after the experience, especially if I am working with the same patient for a few days. I make my own Log. I use my memory to add up observations, but it goes beyond this. It seems like a déjà vu experience.

◊ Yes and no. The memory is there, on tap, available if needed; but it does not predominate. It is the background. The foreground is the wholeness flowing through and being *present now.*

◊ Memory helps, but Therapeutic Touch is more of a unitive experience.

In the next set of statements, it can be seen that time is truly relative, that its meaning is dependent upon the reality to which one refers. The question is stated:

6. *Does any change occur in your sense of time—for instance, does time speed up or slow down?*

◊ Not aware.

◊ Time seemed speeded up here—a lot of internal changes and growth in a short amount of time.

◊ Time speeds up. I am unaware that a half-hour has passed—it seems like five minutes.

◊ Yes. Seems to slow down—that is, time has passed more quickly than I would estimate.

◊ I perceive time slowing down, perhaps because I slow myself down in clearing myself in preparation for the experience.

◊ When I can center and slow down physiologically and emotionally, time seems to become less critical—so I guess it slows down. Anxiety acts to speed it up again, however.

◊ Time slows down, but it does not seem to matter.

◊ Definitely feel time almost stopping for moments and generally slowing down. I feel myself attempting to *hold back* the time in order to absorb as many thoughts and feelings as possible.

◊ Sometimes it stops.

◊ I am not aware of any change in time sense. I am not aware of time.

◊ Have done both. Sometimes I have done this for what seemed like an eternity, only to find that only two minutes or so has passed. Several other times, I have done TT for an "instant" and then have found that five to ten minutes have actually passed.

◊ I am living in the present and not thinking of time. When I think back, time has passed very quickly.

◊ Time does not seem relevant. It doesn't really seem to pass or even exist during the healing.

◊ Time doesn't seem to exist. After the healing act, I'm not sure how much time has passed. It is a much shorter amount of time than I would guess because it seems that a lot has happened. I guess, in that case, that time seems to pass by more slowly.

◊ Time does not exist in the ordinary sense. It is as if one were in a hushed clearing that is both "now" and yet changes. Once I become aware of time again, I am out of the TT state.

◊ At times—if I am centered and compassionate—time sense disappears.

7. *What sense of identity have you—that is, what role do you perceive yourself enacting?*

◊ A student role: I am in unfamiliar waters with waterwings and have a long way to go. Feel as though I've been given enough to float along with for a while, but the depth is awesome.

◊ Right now I am sort of unsure of my role. I am fully cured of doubt that I can indeed be of help to people in need. It's a matter of focusing and transcending the literal, plain, and unadorned pragmatic dimensions of life (does that make sense?).

◊ I perceive myself as an ordinary woman who has always been interested in nursing and in helping people feel better. I do not feel confident in thinking of myself as healer yet, but I would like to. Developing more fully as a woman and giving to each and every person I meet.

◊ Open, friendly, loving; mother, wife, nurse-healer.

◊ As one who can help to alleviate suffering.

◊ During the Assessment, I feel as if I'm just feeling as I would at any other time in order to learn more about something. During healing, I try to remember to be a channel, and sometimes I am, because the energy I feel surprises me. Sometimes, though, when I try to feel energy, I realize that I am tapping into my own energy because I feel a bit nauseated.

◊ As being a human channel.

◊ A channel—unoriginal, but true!

◊ A channel, nothing special, nothing else.

◊ I'm aware that I can feel without actually touching and get acquainted with a body without speech.

◊ A teacher's role—being able to share with others how to maintain a level of wellness and to be responsible for oneself. Also, helping ill people live their lives more comfortably. A tool.

◊ I see myself as trying to help the patient by being a vehicle through which energy can go to the patient in whatever way he or she can use it.

◊ Identity—simple, natural opening up and reaching out to humankind, to growth, and to sharing.

◊ A channel, definitely, for the universal power of wholeness. I am certain it is not "I" who does it, and thus, for the first time this year, I am not tired by it. But I am an *aligned* channel who also translates the wholeness by knowing where to put my hands.

◊ I perceive myself as having something to share, and it gives me satisfaction to feel I can be involved physically with another person's life. It gives me a sense of usefulness that I could never acquire by being a competent accountant, salesperson, and so on.

◊ I see myself trusting my beliefs enough to risk criticism. It feels very good.

◊ That of an explorer.

◊ I perceive myself only as a very real human person returning and giving to others the lessons I have learned—the experiences of love, compassion, being cared for—having myself been in the "same place as others who are now troubled." A return of love and energy for all the gifts of love I have had and now have in my life. My way of thanking God for the gift of life, of being alive.

◊ It's a nice identity because it's natural. It's not different than other living things. This identity is a common denominator.

◊ It seems to me that I have a good sense of identity, and I'd call it a strong sense of identity (though not as a "strong ego"). I feel I'm using myself as an instrument, and, while I'm in control and doing what I want to be doing, I'm really focusing all of my attention on the healee and on the process. If I can learn to use myself as a healer, it will be very gratifying. If I can let the power flow through me, I think I'll feel that it's a wonderful accomplishment. I think I'll feel both proud and humble.

The role of healer is a many faceted one. One of the significant characteristics of the mature healer is a confidence in the healing reality. This reality reflects a natural state that, when we can touch it, serves to allow us to quietly put aside the persona, the mask we wear in public, and to be responsible for our own full stature as Man. This freedom reaches quite deeply into one's being, as is indicated by the answers to the next question:

8. *Are there significant changes in your evaluative and cognitive processes—that is, do you think in a different way during the Therapeutic Touch process than you do ordinarily?*

◊ I have to concentrate and repeatedly return to centering myself. That, together with sensing the energy flows, eliminates most other thoughts.

◊ The quality of thought has more care and is apt to be less negative.

◊ Things that were previously small are becoming more significant and meaningful.

◊ I think I perceive with greater clarity during and just after TT.

◊ I'm a lot more open-minded since being introduced to TT. I used to be a gung-ho "scientific method" addict—I recognized that some people benefited from meditation, belief in energy fields, and so on, but I never was brave enough to let myself try it. Now I find that the experiment was on me, and I have changed without benefit of a "scientific method."

◊ I feel slowed down when I do an Assessment. I feel my thought processes are sharper at that time. I think that the quality of my thoughts have improved.

◊ Thought processes seem to spring from intuitional insight rather than rationality.

◊ My thought processes are slower as I grope to realize and organize thoughts at a deeper level.

◊ I constantly grow in my appreciation of all things around or within me.

◊ My thoughts are more deliberative and contemplative after healing, and it seems that any thoughts I have during healing do not have a place; rather, they are interfering with the process and come from another "place" in my mind.

◇ Feelings feel "right," more so than analysis. I feel my sensitivity increase, and I am able to tune in more quickly to my perceptions.

◇ Yes, my mental processes are more focused than usual; the on-going evaluation is more intense than it usually is.

◇ Yes, I think that instead of just looking at one part of a situation, I'm looking at the total process. Also, I'm trying to feel besides just looking with my eyes.

◇ My thoughts are more meaningful, as though I finally found all the edge pieces to my puzzle and now can put the middle parts together. Yes, thoughts flow rapidly . . . very freely, peacefully . . . as in a meditative state. Cognitive processes seem to slip into the background, or maybe they become secondary to a more intuitive sense.

◇ Thoughts stop—and intuitions, images, and impressions take over.

◇ At my best, there are few thoughts and, occasionally, none.

◇ Sharpened, focused, and therefore slowed down. At the same time, quicker, and there is more self-confidence in the judgment.

◇ I feel it primarily as a broadening experience that gives some form to what were previously only murky waters. I was aware of this, but I had never investigated it seriously or systematically. My cognitive processes are well developed—sometimes they just need some help in an appropriate direction.

◇ I think in a very organized manner as I have this internal conversation with myself.

◇ The process seems different because it is fast, all-or-none, and *irreversible,* whereas the more familiar analytical process is methodical, step-by-step, and *reversible.* I think that the reversible and irreversible differences are important to me in TT. Yes, that is one significant difference between the two processes.

In these answers, we come in touch with something of the quality of the healing reality, a state of consciousness where a sense of immediacy prevails: You know, and you know that you know. However, it is not the case that you do not know how you know. You have permitted yourself to let down the culture-bound barriers, and, in a conscious manner, you have been willing to expose yourself to an alternative mode of cognition. It is a challenging frontier to scale, and it does take courage to test oneself against an interior reality that has just begun to be understood in this new, more permissive age. It is a reality in which each individual is the sole judge of the validity and reliability of his or her perceptions; this judgment must nevertheless be honed to a fine edge against the touchstones of other realities by which Man also judges.

The final question in this series further explores the healer's perception of him- or herself:

9. *How do you perceive your body image—that is, what feedback do you get from the movements, postures, and energetic flow of your body?*

◊ I do not believe that my body image is good—I feel a lot of negative thoughts about it. I think that with time and increased awareness this will improve.

◊ I had not considered my body image in this before. Of course, it feels better to be in a comfortable position. I will pay more attention to this in the future.

◊ I have yet to learn a lot about my own body's perceptions. I need practice.

◊ At this point, I am only becoming aware that I possess these things! I feel a need to study and experiment a great deal more.

◊ I focus on what my hands tell me. I find that if I am "crossed" or "kinked," I perceive very little in my hands. I then pick up anxiety from anxious clients easily and have to discharge it consciously. At these times, I am also aware that I feel a tightness in my chest.

◊ I relate to a healthy, fit, energetic body.

◊ I have a good perception of my body image. I feel that I am accomplishing something good, and this gives me internal energy.

◊ My body feels in harmony and seems more like an instrument to me, for the energy flows through me more strongly during the Therapeutic Touch process. I am not very conscious of my body except in that way, unless I've gotten into an uncomfortable position.

◇ I am aware of feedback from my body—it tells me when I am uncomfortable, for example. I had previously ignored this.

◇ I don't seem to think much about my body posture except when it's in a posture in which I cannot reach someone's body; then I move.

◇ I don't always have a comfortable posture, but my movements are developing into positions of more ease. I feel that I have to work more on the development of a flow to my body movements.

◇ I become very sensitive to how I move my body, whether I'm putting myself into an awkward, stressful position or if I am moving with grace and good body mechanics. If my body is well grounded and relaxed, I feel stronger and more intent on what I am doing.

◇ Postures which may be uncomfortable at other times can be maintained longer. Also, circulation seems improved, my hands and feet are warmer, energy flow feels more free, and movement often becomes quite subtle and soft.

◇ When I feel uncomfortable, I feel I can work on this and have the control to remove this discomfort. I am also aware that I have a natural flow of energy when I allow it to flow and do not block it.

◇ My body is mostly comfortable and energetic, but still needs more work.

◇ Not from movements or postures, but I particularly enjoy it when my neck and shoulders feel free. I take that as a sign of good energy flow from me to the healee.

◇ I feel my own energy and I feel I can activate it.

◇ I like my body and listen to its signals to me and try to decipher what it needs. I also feel that I have command over it to be used as I see fit—in this case, as an instrument.

◇ More relaxed, but conscious of more power.

◇ My body is more *alive,* because it works in its entirety! I feel as though my body is working in unison. My whole body is united.

◇ I seem to stand or kneel straighter, as if allowing a more direct flow of energy—and yet I am more relaxed.

- ◊ At times I feel warm and drawn up straight, and kind of revitalized.
- ◊ A positive feeling related, it seems, to relaxation and a centering of my energies.
- ◊ I get increased feedback when I am relaxed and centered.
- ◊ A sense of relaxation, warmth, freedom from discomfort. I cease to think of my body in parts, but as a continuous flowing river of warm energy, with my arms the extension of self to connect with other people or objects—the rest of my world.
- ◊ I feel comfortable with the concept that I am a channel—energy moves in and out of me without a need to use it as power.
- ◊ Hushed stillness and harmony. The heat or tingling in my hands is joyful, and I have an image of my own stillness, the patient's stillness, and a universal stillness.
- ◊ Usually I feel relaxed, but with vigor and a sense that I am doing my work—that it has great meaning in my life and that the next years will be a real deepening process for me.
- ◊ My body image is more together, but my vocabulary for describing the healing touch is very limited. I need to work on articulating precisely what happens and what is felt. We need a new language for this.

This last sentence, I believe, is very significant: We do need a new language to describe this unique experience into the inner spaces of self, a space which our bodies can translate only the most subtle intimations of for us.

The recording of a personal journal over an extended period of time is one way to catch these fleeting impressions based on experiential data. Let us, therefore, once again take a look over the shoulders of other persons who are practicing Therapeutic Touch and get a closer glimpse of the healing reality as seen through their eyes, in their journals. In order to provide an opportunity for you to relate more closely to their experiences, I will present the beginning entries in the approximate order of your experiences while you were reading *The Therapeutic Touch: How to Use the Hands to Help or to Heal,* and then enlarge the scope of material so that you can get a broader idea of how other persons have applied Therapeutic Touch.

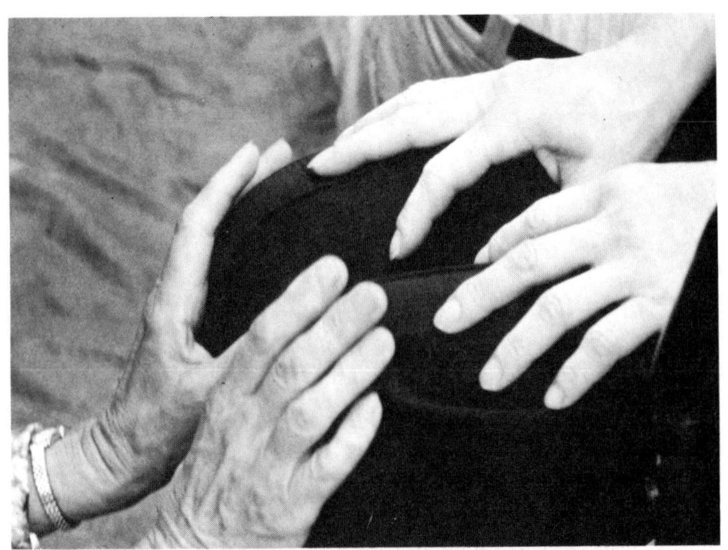

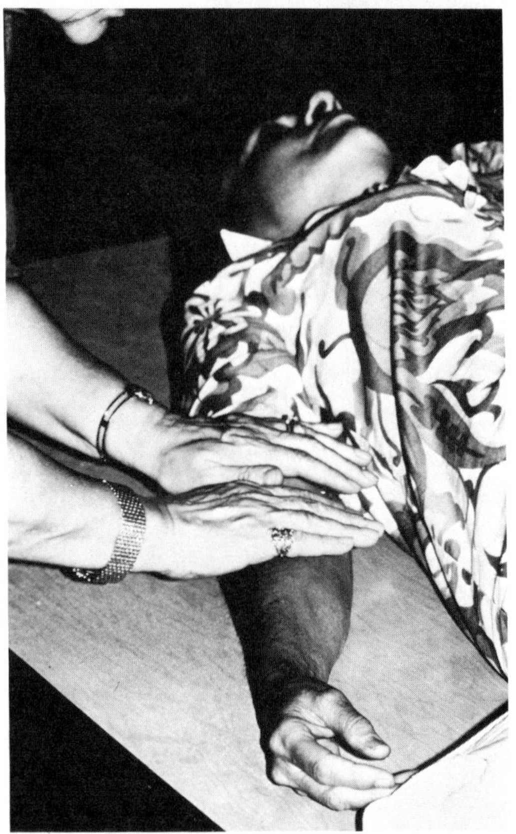

Practicing Therapeutic Touch.

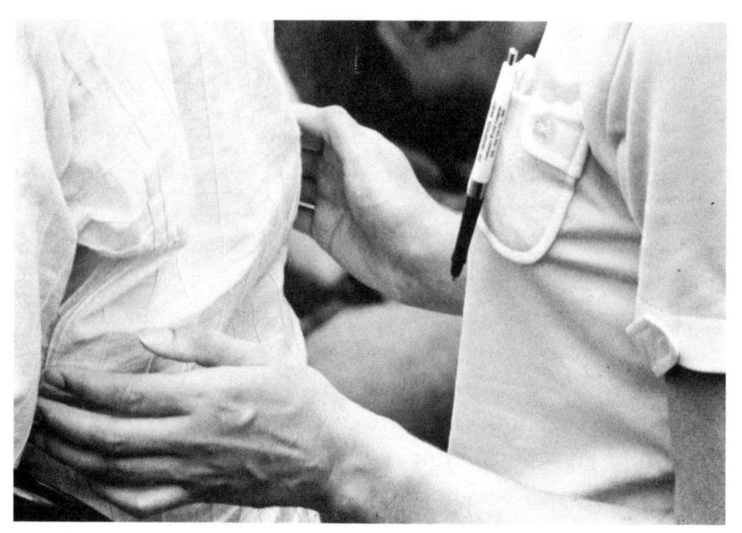

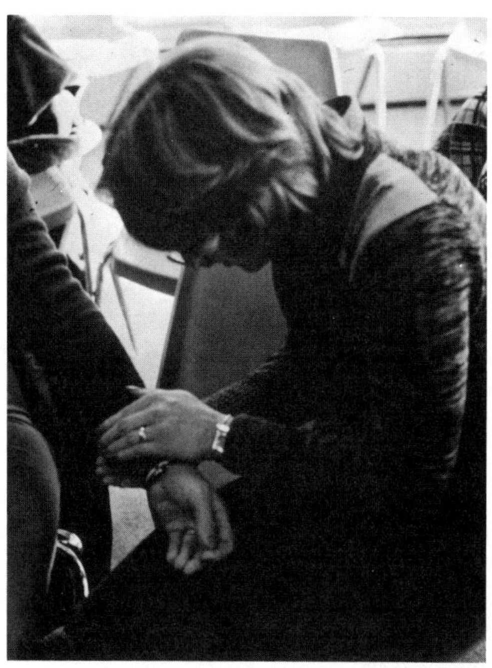

Practicing Therapeutic Touch.

INTENTIONALITY

Interestingly, much of what we have discussed in class and what I am now doing are things that I had done before. There was, of course, one big difference: Now I was very aware of what I was doing. In the past, many of the things I did when caring for people were frequently done almost automatically. For example, if I were caring for an infant, I would usually do the same thing with each infant in my care—that is, I would pick up the child for a while after feeding or caring for it and then put it back in a crib, usually lying on its side or stomach. Now, I notice what I am doing with infants, and I do not respond to each in the same way. As I approach an infant, I find myself centering, so that the primary concern is the child and what he or she is communicating to me. Out of this communication and subsequent assessment, I decide how I can best intervene in the interests of this little one.

M.O.

MOTIVATION

Having to come to grips with my motivations for wanting to help led me to examine certain aspects of myself that I had previously waved aside. I began to see that this was necessary, although it was not particularly inviting for me. This developed into a passage, an emergence for me. It brought me in touch with symbols that had lain forgotten for many years. My original image of a nurse was as a rescuer—I would save my sister. Interwoven with this was the memory that she, too, had had the capacity to sense the need for help, and to help. I remembered my realization that the grieving process held within it a potential for growth—repatterning—and that it shared commonalities with Therapeutic Touch in the preparation of this repatterning. I had to come to grips with myself regarding *why* I wanted to do Therapeutic Touch—not to be a sensation, or to exercise power and control over others, but to approach a human being as one who wanted to share and to help.

M.S.

ACCEPTANCE OF SELF

I've come to an acceptance of my own potential; I can accept Therapeutic Touch and the role I have come to play in it. I feel that the path that I took was inevitable for me; however, I could not begin to see myself as a link until I was absolutely sure of myself. My fear or hesitation in relation to Therapeutic Touch was that I would abuse it. I had to learn more about myself as a person and as a nurse and develop a personal philosophy for its use. It all seemed to jell somehow. What initially hadn't seemed to make much sense served as a basis for my moving on to experience Therapeutic Touch. Being able to mentally construct a union with the totality of man–environment lent me a sense of harmony, of well-being. I had to accept my own humanness in order to share it with others:

> The joy is in the change, the process, not the attainment.[1]

M.S.

HAND EXERCISES

As I reread my journal about my experiences with Therapeutic Touch, I find that there were many interesting and "unusual" experiences and happenings, but somehow, in retrospect, I am less inclined to label them as "unusual." As I grow experientially and become more aware, even the unexplainable happenings are no longer bizarre; they are simply *new* experiences.

I would like to share with you some of the new experiences and feelings that I have had during the past few months as I learned and experienced Therapeutic Touch.

My first experience with Therapeutic Touch was on the first day of class. I was instructed to hold my hand palm to palm and then move them a few inches apart. By doing so, I became aware of something, some feeling—a field force or energy—between my hands. I saw my student/

[1] Bob Tobin, *Space Time and Beyond* (New York: E.P. Dutton and Co., 1975), p. 116.

learner role as that of someone who had much to learn about this new field of study. I was conscious of my own awareness of the experience, and I was also very willing to let my mind be open to whatever there was to experience in spite of the *avant garde* nature of the subject. I was conscious of my hands and the tingling I felt in my fingers. I felt the sense of pressure of the energy field between them. The hands, which I had thought of all my life as appendages, took on new meaning. I was aware of them for the first time as extensions of my mind.

Later that same night, at a seminar, I experienced that same sensation of an energy field as I sat next to someone. I sensed that the energy was being radiated between us and from us. The two bodies close together created the same energy field as the two hands close together. Now I realized that my body was an extension of my mind.

M.A.M.

One night, I was practicing Therapeutic Touch and decided to hold my boyfriend's hands (not telling him what I was doing). I felt heat coming from the *chakras* of my hand, but it wasn't as much as I had felt in class. I attempted to send my energy across the junction of space between our hands. He did not acknowledge any sensation, but I observed an occasional twitch in his thumb, so I stopped and went over to my dog, who was lying on her belly, head up.

I tried an Assessment, but felt no difference. I then placed my hand at the back of her neck without touching her, about an inch away, and left it there. Shortly, she sighed and put her head down, apparently to get more comfortable. Soon after, she began to twitch occasionally, down to and including her tail, and then she went to sleep.

I concluded that something must have happened due to the similarity of twitches in response to my attempts to transfer energy. So I went back to my guy, who was dozing by this time, but not fully asleep, and began an Assessment from his neck to his pelvic area. I thought I felt a greater concentration of energy in the area of his stomach, just below the esophageal sphincter, so I left my hand there for a little while without touching him, waiting for a response. When I thought I felt a difference, although it was mild, I tried to move the energy towards his feet. He responded, half unconscious, "H'm that feels good," but I wasn't touching him. The time involved was only about three minutes. As soon as I stopped, he mumbled: "Thank you. I feel so much more relaxed," and immediately fell asleep.

M.O.S.

DOWSING RODS

I tried the dowsing rods with Jenny. She's a short person, and so I didn't think they would have time to cross and uncross again. Also, she has cystic fibrosis, and I figured that that would affect things. However, I went over her body very slowly, and they did cross in exactly the five areas of her body as they should.

M.K.

This is my first journal, as it took me a long time to put down the things that happened to me, because I wanted to be sure of myself.

With the help of a friend, I practiced the exercises we did in class, such as those with the dowsing rods. As you demonstrated them in class there was no question in my mind when I saw the rods cross over the forehead, neck, solar plexus, the knees, and the ankles. But when I was going to do it on my friend, she expressed doubt and said, "These rods won't cross unless you influence them in some way." As I passed them over her supine body, they did cross exactly where predicted, and I was aware that I didn't help them in any way. In order to convince her, I let her do the same thing on me, and it happened to me as it had to her. Her doubt vanished with her amazement, and she remarked, "I sure felt the increase in the energy fields as the rods crossed. It's great!"

N.P.

To continue with my experiences in reference to the dowsing rods, I find that as I progress with my pregnancy, my field integrity is altering drastically. In my first trimester, the dowsing rods crossed at all the five designated points. Now, in the second semester, they go "haywire" over my solar plexus area.

C.B.

USE OF COTTON TO FACILITATE HEALING

Sunday afternoon, my husband returned home from bowling with the children because our ten-year-old son, Bill, had a very swollen right thumb. When I examined his thumb, I found it to be approximately two and a half times the size of the left thumb, hot, and very red, with a small cut of about three-eighths of an inch on the back of his hand (a leftover from the previous week when he had cut himself, had washed the wound, and had never told us about it). In addition, he also had extensive soft tissue swelling of two-thirds of his hand. I immediately began hot soaks, but by evening it was apparent that a lymphangitis was developing. A call to the pediatrician, and Bill was started on a ten-day course of treatment with a broad spectrum antibiotic. The swelling, redness, and purulent drainage subsided, but a firm thickness persisted, so that by the end of the ten days, both the pediatrician and I were concerned that an osteomyelitis might be developing.

It was then that I decided to use Therapeutic Touch. Because of my emotional involvement with the child and the difficult time I was having learning to center (I had never meditated previously), I decided that I would use the cotton which I had energized to facilitate the healing process.

That day, I picked Bill up at school, and as we drove home, I asked about his thumb and told him that I had something new and special that would make it well. He asked if it would be like his other medications and then asked persistently what it was called. Finally, deciding not to wait until we reached home, I said: "It's called Therapeutic Touch." His response, in a very accepting manner, was: "Oh, that . . . Goodee . . ee! . . . (giggle) . . . I'm going to be part of an experiment!" I gave him the cotton, which I had with me, and told him to wrap it around his thumb for a while.

After about five minutes, I asked Bill how the cotton felt. He smiled and said, "It feels nice . . . and . . . soft." My thought was one of disappointment; so, I thought, everyone thinks cotton is soft. Bill continued: ". . . and warm." I still felt a measure of disappointment. ". . . And every once in a while it feels like a tickle in my whole thumb." Ah-ha! there it was! Needless to say, I felt delighted.

Thereafter, on the fifteen-minute ride to and from school, and again in the evening, Bill held the cotton I had energized around his thumb and always described his sensations in a similar fashion. In less than a week, approximately 90% of the thickness, which had persisted for almost two weeks previously, was gone. Since that time, the remaining thickness has disappeared and with it my fear of osteomyelitis.

During this experience, I was amazed at how easily the child accepted the idea and believed it would help. I am sure that this occurred because he had heard me talking about it in a realistic and enthusiastic manner. His calm acceptance reinforced and enhanced the healing milieu, I am sure.

L.L.H.

CENTERING

To my understanding, Therapeutic Touch starts with learning to be centered. The first time I tried the technique, I wondered: "Will I know the feeling? How will it happen? What will I feel?" But I needn't have worried; it happened as naturally as breathing. I began by consciously relaxing, by feeling totally open to the natural flow of the universe.

> It is well documented that the meditative state itself produces distinct and positive physiological changes. . . .[2]

A deep, calm wave flowed in on the first breath. It flowed more deeply on the second, and on the third breath I felt a stir, a whirring deep within my being—so deep, and tucked away behind a cryptic, visceral place I'd never known or felt before. A secret place once somnolent, dormant, was now awakened. I was aware of my breath moving in me, but somehow beyond the space of my lungs, and I was acutely aware of my very being and my existence with the universe. I was, as Pelletier says: "pervaded with the overwhelming and joyous knowledge that all of existence is a unity and that I was one with it and one and the same as all else about me."[3]

I could feel with each inspiration and expiration the flow of all that existed within me. It seemed to be an innate, but dimly remembered, knowledge, a natural flow from the source of one's being; and the beauty of the implicit pattern and organization of it all was like a dazzling truth revealed. I was in awe of my centering experience and anxious to try channeling this energy through Therapeutic Touch. I was self-conscious, uncertain, but I knew I had to try.

E.S.

[2] Kenneth Pelletier, *Mind as Healer, Mind as Slayer* (New York: Dell Publishing Co., 1977), p. 209.

[3] Pelletier, *op. cit.*, p. 226.

My main concern in the beginning was to get enough information and knowledge so that I could engage in Therapeutic Touch from a sound, solid base. Throughout the readings, the class lectures, and the classroom experience, I kept hearing "center," "centering," and "from your center," and I realized its importance. As I began to experience "centering," images became quite vivid. At first, the images were of light rays and warmth. I related this to my own physical energy system both within me and flowing through and beyond me. I am, indeed, an open system, continuously exchanging matter and energy with my environment. I realized this and came to understand that this energy exchange is a natural and normal process.

P.H.

Often I would sit in my car before entering a patient's house, knowing that I was not ready to go in. I would sit quietly for a few minutes so that when I entered the house I would be able to become attuned to the patient, to partially sense his or her world as if it were my own.

M.S.

CENTERING WHILE BEING A HEALEE

By the seventh week of class, I was convinced that centering myself altered my state of consciousness. It was at this time that I experienced a terrible backache, and Therapeutic Touch was performed on me at my request. With me as the subject, Dee Krieger and a classmate put their hands over me. As they did so, I felt myself become centered. . . . As I concentrated on the warmth from their hands, I could "feel" myself sitting, so to speak, in the center of the field they created. With my eyes closed, the perception of the experience was enhanced. I could "see" the field that they had created as they moved their hands down my body, even though they had yet to make physical contact with me.

I wrote of this experience in Nursymbolese and later analyzed it. During the experience, I became aware of the flow of energy between us as a mutual, simultaneous interaction. Although I know that I was receiving energy from the healers and that the healers were attempting to reduce my pain and bring my body back into equilibrium, I felt energy being taken from me as well. Perhaps this was "negative" energy in the form of pain, but I felt an enmeshing of our energy fields, as if there was a mutual energy exchange in the attempt to bring my field back into balance. Later, as I felt the heat from Dee's touch with one hand on my shoulder and the other at my back, I felt only the in-put of her energy to me, not a simultaneous loss from me. An equilibrium was established. . . . I do not remember exactly when my back stopped hurting, but the next day I discovered that I was without pain.

M.A.M.

AN EFFECT OF NOT CENTERING

A nurse in the operating room complained of periodic migraine. I offered to help her. In between cases, I applied Therapeutic Touch techniques. After each encounter, I asked her if she noticed anything unusual happening. Each time she said, "Nothing." On my part, as the healer, I also did not feel anything. This is one of the cases that was a failure.

Where did I fail? I kept asking myself. Recollecting the previous cases, I finally came upon the following answer. To begin with, the place was not conducive to the healing process. The room that we chose was always full of people coming and going. There was no peace or quiet. The patient and I were not relaxed. When I put my hands near the afflicted area, I could feel tension in my fingers. I was not at ease, and in my concern over this, I failed to center myself and thereby failed to help my friend.

V.G.C.

THE ASSESSMENT

I did have one very encouraging experience. I kept finding a difference in temperature on the foot of a patient and was able to ask him if there had ever been anything wrong with his foot. I had known him for several days, and we had built up a trusting friendship. He seemed a little embarrassed and said that he did suffer from some form of gout and that he had been in pain for the past two days but had feared to mention it since he did not want anyone to think that he had a disease that "drinkers get." I assured him that such was not the case and told him that I would send the doctor to him so that medical treatment could be begun.

The only difficult part of this episode was when he asked me how I knew about his foot. He wanted to know if I could see something in his face. "Do I look like a drinker?" he asked.

R.F.

I arrived home, and my husband complained of pain in his lower back, a recurrent problem. During my Assessment, I noted a cool area over his right lower back. I finished the Assessment and returned to the area for confirmation. I was puzzled that I had felt a difference only on the one side and told my husband about my Assessment. I was quite surprised when he informed me that the pain was only in his lower right back.

S.R.

VISUALIZATIONS

In the beginning of my experience, I was not conscious of any imagery, but, in retrospect, there was always the gray-white, mottled, ever-changing enveloping atmosphere that I saw. I gradually came to recognize that there were differences in the patterning, though. The painful injections and the crying infant presented a dark and gray pattern to me. I was also able to perceive heat over the injection site. I don't know why, but one day recently I became aware that these patterned fields were ever-changing and that they seemed to be a kind of visualization of an arrangement of cells or molecules. The darker I perceived the field, the more distress was perceived by the healee. These areas of discomfort did not necessarily correlate with the medical opinion, but it did with the client's opinion.

This awareness of patterning is recent to me and needs further investigation and correlation to events, but it is the way I perceive the field to date. I feel that this is a clue to what for me may be a way of assessment, but it needs practice.

N.O.

CREATIVE IMAGERY

The experiential lab in creative imagery was familiar to me. As a child, I used to entertain myself with this type of experience at night. Then, the images seemed brighter and more explosive in nature.

The experience in class was more subtle. . . . During the experience, I was aware of a reddish warm color, a sun type image, moving across a screen. Masses and forms moving into the center, merging and pulling apart. Fluidic images, like clouds moving across the sky. Every now and then something lighter moved in and then moved out and away. It was a rhythmic image, like the sea when it's calm. Then there was a feeling of moving forward, passing through. The background became darker, with lighter images. When the images were moving, I could see them sometimes as in stop-action photography, as though they were falling. When an image moved, it rolled in. The images presented themselves as though I had tunnel vision directly ahead of me. Again, a change to alternating light and dark images moving across, very soft, dim, and fuzzy. It was similar to when you look hard in darkness: There is still a vibrancy, even though it's dark. The images collided and then went off in other directions.

My readings have led me to interpret the experience depicted above as a moving toward an individual awareness in which I am a participant.

> The symbol is not an allegory and not a sign, but an image of a content that largely transcends consciousness.[4]

I can only relate to this experience as an emerging consciousness—my examination of a coexisting reality.

M.S.

[4] Jolande Jacobi, *The Psychology of C.G. Jung* (New York: Pantheon Books, 1973), p. 97.

THINK BLUE

On this particular day in class, we were told to center and then to think of various colors, such as blue, bright yellow, and green. We visualized other objects and then we were told to think of someone we love, to try to get an idea of where that person was at that time and of what he or she was doing.

I pictured a very dear friend. We had had an argument a week prior, and since then, there had been no verbal communication. At 5:30 P.M. (later that day), he called. He had a very pleasant attitude and was very loving. Three days later, I got up enough courage to ask him where he was on that particular day. He told me he had been in his office. I asked if he was wearing a gray suit then. He said he was. I went further to ask him if he was thinking about me at that time, and he said that he was. I told him that all my energies were directed at him at that time. He became very scared. I discussed with him the class I am attending, but that didn't help—he still acted scared. So I began touching him, which had a tremendous calming effect.

He is still skeptical, but that's all right!

P.R.

THE PHENOMENOLOGY OF THERAPEUTIC TOUCH

After consciously deciding that I do indeed desire to help, I assess my own energy field in order to determine whether I have the needed energy to do so. If so, I go deeper into the centering process, which somehow has already begun during the period of self-assessment. A different or altered state of consciousness occurs, which seems to make necessary adjustments in my field boundaries.

Finally, I am ready to reach out and assess the person in need of healing. Although it would appear that I do this primarily through my hands, this is only part of the story: Interestingly, my whole field is actively "listening" and picking up information from the healee's field. The heat, the cold, and the tingling in the palms of my hands seem to be merely symbolic of what is really going on in this holistic phenomenon! Primarily guided by my hands (which in turn are guided by my whole field), I begin to will or think and direct energy towards the healee with the intention of facilitating a free flow of energy throughout his or her entire field.

I am more comfortable when I sense his or her energy flowing in a circular fashion. Sometimes, it seems, I try to "speed up" the process of the flow without trying to influence the direction. However, if I "pick up" any constrictions or any sense of blockage (which, for some reason, I sense in the area of my solar plexus), I tend to try to consciously direct the energy through the constricted area.

Most often, I find that I "give" and direct energy through my left hand and "cast off" the feeling of congested or static energy with my right hand. However, I have had the experience a few times of using both hands to transmit the energy, and there was none to "cast off"; it was as if the person were a sponge, soaking up all the energy I could give.

Time perception is definitely altered; there is a speeding up or timelessness about it. The more intensely I am involved, the more the experience is lifted out of time as we ordinarily experience it. What has always amazed me is the sudden and definite *STOP!* that comes unmistakably and is unannounced, although recently I seem to be becoming more sensitive and able to "tune in" to the gentle whisper that just precedes it and says: "almost . . . almost."

Throughout the whole interaction, I remain very aware of the integrity of my own field boundaries. Although this serves as a protection, according to Bennett, it is also a property of wholeness:

> Wholeness is noted to be omnipresent but relative . . . gradations of wholeness . . . are determined by the extent or degree to which a given object is itself and does not merge into something that is not itself.[5]

As soon as I get the message to stop, I do just that, saying: "OK, that's it!" and saying it in such a way that it really seems to carry with it my last spurt of energy to the other person's field.

The feeling I have afterwards is usually one of a sense of accomplishment—strangely enough, this happens whether or not the person

[5] J.G. Bennett, *The Foundations of a Natural Philosophy* (London: Hodder and Stroughton, 1956), p. 6.

reports that he has been helped. There is a certain joy in simply knowing that I have done everything I possibly could to facilitate healing. Of course, I feel even better when the other person is actually helped or healed!

M.E.K.

When in the process of healing, I experienced repetitive patterns of sensations, with different intensities for each experience. Whenever I began to "heal" someone, I consciously took a deep breath and relaxed or centered myself. I concentrated on my hands to pick up differences in temperature or other sensations; but with experience, I find this to be less deliberate and easier to accomplish. Sometimes, I've found myself to be spontaneously passing my hands slowly over a painful arm or swollen area as if I knew the swelling or "congestion" had to be relieved or set free. In these situations, moreover, I've found that modulating my energy to "think blue" to be very helpful in dissipating the heat from the area.

E.G.

During the act of Therapeutic Touch, my perception of the healee is such that I feel an access to, and increased understanding of, the person as a whole. As for myself, I feel more together, part of an harmonic flow. Emotionally, I am unafraid, and I have a sense of shared optimism with the healee; neither nervousness nor anxiety has a place in this reality. The focus is on the healee as a fellow human being, on the sharing of an inner-directed energy.

M.S.

In reference to my pregnancy, I find my field involuting more and more on a daily basis. In this context, the more my field "shrinks," the less able I am to be a therapeutic healer. I find that it has become very difficult for me to center myself, as well as to open my field to another in order that he or she may use the potential energies that I may have available to share with them.

C.S.B.

During the healing act of Therapeutic Touch, my hands are my eyes and ears. They can see light and dark; they feel heat and cold; they hear the waves, the beeps, the blips. They can sense "clogs," "stuffinesses," or "blockages." They can pick up rates and rhythms, fast and slow, smooth or jerky. Oddly enough, time loses all meaning during Therapeutic Touch; time is transcended by the healing process itself.

My mind's eye, which seems to be located in the palms of my hands, has great powers of concentration. During Therapeutic Touch, I can sense and more fully feel my patient in a way that is not possible with mere monitoring of vital signs. It is here that another seemingly paradoxical situation exists. While "in touch" with the healee, I am also aware of and in contact with the environment—that is, I feel just as involved with the people and things around me when I do Therapeutic Touch as I am at any other time. When I am properly centered for Therapeutic Touch, environmental noises do not usually disturb me. My own "inner noises" are more quiet, and somehow this makes it possible for me to accept external noise. The enhanced quality of patient perception during Therapeutic Touch seems to be matched with an enhanced quality of environmental perception.

The heightened sense of patient and environment follows in the path of my overall heightened sense of self. I feel a greater potential for a clearer and more true sense of healing during Therapeutic Touch. Within the healee-self-environment system, I perceive myself as a catalytic instrument involved in the healing process—a sort of guided beam of energy whose intent is that the path to health can be followed more readily.

P.Y.

I observe my client walking towards me. He is tall and lean, with stooped shoulders and a slow, plodding gait. His appearance is neat, conservative, almost meticulous. He glances briefly at me, maintains eye contact only for a moment, and then sits heavily in the chair. His hands are clasping and gripping the arms of the chair. His face appears tired, tense, and drawn. When I ask him how he is doing, he replies: "Terrible."

The ambient temperature in the room is cool. I inhale deeply, feeling the coolness of the air rush in the tip of my nostrils. I continue focusing on the air going through my nasal passages and into my chest. In . . . out. . . . I am breathing slowly and deeply. I gradually become aware of a large, dark abyss located in the center of my very being and swelling within me. There is nothing present now in the environment but my client and me. It is as if we are meeting and are suspended in space-time.

Without speaking, I start the Assessment at the top of his head and work downwards. I work slowly, methodically, searching for change. I proceed carefully over the client's body. He has begun to relax now, too, with his hands resting comfortably at his sides. His breathing is slow and regular.

After completing the Assessment, I return my hands to the back of his neck, where I had felt heat on the initial scanning. At this time, the heat seems to me to be even more intense, and I act to dissipate this bound energy. I place my hands over the area and feel the transfer of heat, which seems to fill up my hands. I shake the heat out of my hands with several flicks of the wrist. This continues for some time, but it is difficult to judge how long. We seem to be caught up in a timelessness.

As the heat gradually dissipates, I reverse the process and focus on my hands. I slip deeper within myself, calling forth positive thoughts of love to direct towards my client. I am looking at my hands. Do they really belong to me? They are tools heavily suspended in midair at the ends of my arms; they almost have an existence outside myself.

Now, I am reaching a new height of awareness. Seeming to soar, I laugh joyously inside of me at the delight I am experiencing. My consciousness is not aware of the healee's separateness. He and I are one, united, composed of flowing energy. It is the height of aliveness, of experiencing my humanness!

The high subsides to a quiet peace within me, and I know that we are through with our interaction at this level. The sounds and colors in the background begin to filter into awareness, but they are not the same as before. They are muffled and soft and rosy. It is a nice place to be, and I feel at one with my world. My client is smiling broadly. He says, "Thank you." His voice is low and hushed. His face is flushed, and the tenseness in his brow has disappeared. His headache is gone. We share the same joy and peace and are at one with the world.

K.W.

Quite a number of the journal entries deal with the process of Therapeutic Touch. In these instances, I was more actively participating in this other reality, trying to understand it and to work with it. My attitude was essentially the same in all cases; it was positive and concerned. I wanted to share what I knew and also to learn more from the experiences. The healees' attitudes were basically open and hopeful. None of them had any tremendous faith in Therapeutic Touch or in me as a healer, but they loved and respected me as a friend and knew that I would never try to manipulate or hurt them.

The two instances of my friends who had bronchitis are very similar, and they are also representative of the interactions I experienced. In each case, I could feel a sensation of heat emanating from localized parts of their bodies. I tried to "push" the heat away, and as I did this I felt a subtle pressure, resembling that of water, building up in front of my hands. At this same time, in each case, my friends felt the congestion inside them flowing out of their bodies. Here again, we can see a relationship between the objective reality and the other reality. Also, in both cases, I eventually perceived a sense of "nothingness." No difference could be noted between their otherness and mine, as though a kind of fusion had occurred, and I thought of the way water always seeks its own level and eventually finds it.

In thinking about these experiences, the water symbol comes to my mind again and again. To me, it means a universal substance and force, fundamental to all living beings and yet owned by none of them.

J.M.

EXPERIENCES DURING THE THERAPEUTIC TOUCH PROCESS

Then I met Adrienne—a totally frustrating experience! She had many problems, mostly psychological, resulting in many psychosomatic symptoms. Many of us tried to reach her, but she carried on a constant monologue of symptoms and demanded analgesics or narcotics frequently. I tried to get her to try meditation, about which she had bought several books, but without success. I felt that she would feel threatened if I suggested Therapeutic Touch, so I just thought about her without otherwise intervening.

Whenever I thought about her, however, I immediately got the sense as though I was pushing against a wall. Not only did I meet resistance, but I felt a pushing back, like waves hitting a solid stone wall and bouncing back. After this encounter, I would have a dull headache, which seemed to worsen if I tried to integrate the experience. Sometimes, I would feel complete exhaustion. Reviewing this experience later, I thought that perhaps I hadn't been feeling well or that I lacked energy.

I tried again two days later; but immediately I began to get a headache, and so I left the room. I didn't try again; however, after reading LeShan's explanation of the negative effect encountered by one of his students, I was better able to integrate this experience.

> In the first [case], the patient actively does not want the healing. This is a clear experience that one of my students in psychic healing has described as ". . . feeling as if you were running into a rubber wall." . . . Put bluntly, it is impossible to "unite" with someone who does not want to unite with you.[6]

N.O.T.

I finally decided to tell a few of my fellow staff members of my first healing experiences. I said, "This is probably just a coincidence, but! . . ." I received a mixed reception. Most of them thought I was crazy. One said, "Maybe you've been going to school too long?" Another, of whom I am very fond, said, "That's the work of the devil!"

That bothered me a great deal. I had thought that I had left most of my regimented parochial schooling behind. Years of training by dedicated nuns had left me with many hang-ups–some good, some bad. I looked up all the "Healings Described in the New Testament" as listed by Dearmer.[7] I could find no suggestion of the devil's work there; rather, I got the distinct feeling that Jesus expected us to have faith in our ability to heal. His disciples did so much healing; a prerequisite seemed to be that they had faith in their ability to heal.

In class the following Thursday, Ann, who is from the Islands, mentioned that her folks used visualization and healing in the Virgin Islands until the missionaries came and told them that it was wrong. It was only now, she said, that she was beginning to see that it was all right again. That seemed to parallel my own experience and made me feel more confident of my own feelings.

Even though I was now gaining a little confidence, I still had the feeling that one had to be a saint, or close to it, in order to heal anyone. Then I read:

> . . . We find no New Testament backing for the view that healings

[6] Lawrence LeShan, *The Medium, The Mystic and The Physicist: Toward a General Theory of the Paranormal* (New York: The Viking Press, 1974), p. 129.

[7] Percy Dearmer, *Body and Soul* (London: Sir Isaac Pitman and Sons, 1909).

> take place to show that a person is a saint. On the contrary, Jesus seems to assume that extraordinary actions will be performed by ordinary . . . men. Moreover, He said that one of the signs that will follow those that believe (not necessarily those who are holy) will be that they will lay hands on the sick, and they will recover.[8]

Wow! How about that? Even me! And for further back-up:

> Although written thousands of years before Christ, the combination of religion and prayer for healing is found in the books of the Ayur-Veda, which deals with medical arts taken from the sacred Vedas, the oldest writings known on the surface of the Earth.[9]

Coupled with all the positive experiences I was hearing about in class, I felt that I had a solid philosophical base, and I felt very good, almost ecstatic, about this.

Although I now feel that the act of healing is supported by my religion, I do not feel the necessity of involving prayer in this act. My feeling seems to be the same as Oskar Estebany's (Mr. E.):

> Though he is a Roman Catholic, a "believer Catholic" as he puts it, Mr. E. says that he does not pray or ask God for help during the laying-on of hands. He believes that his ability is God-given and, having acknowledged this, he feels it is his duty to get on with his work without badgering God for constant reassurances.[10]

Presently, my healing experiences do not involve prayer. I seem to need the assurance that it is all right with God, but I do not actively seek his help. I seem to feel that I do have a beginning ability to direct this energy, and the direction comes from my own intense desire to help.

J.M.

Currently, I find my mental focus shifting inwards, self questioning self in terms of the depth and intensity of my caring. Do I care *enough*

[8] Lori J. Zefron, "The History of the Laying-on of Hands in Nursing," *Nursing Forum 14:* (1975), 354.

[9] Zefron, *op. cit.,* 355.

[10] David M. Rorvik, "The Healing Hands of Mr. E.," *Esquire 81:* (1974), 159.

in the healing situation to be effective? Can I really "tune in" and helpfully affect the other's field? Thinking about this phenomenon of healing, I realize that I cannot assess the healing attempt because I have been reluctant to notify *and* involve the healee in the Therapeutic Touch process and consequently have not operationalized the process fully. I suspect that open communication is inherent to therapeutic energy exchange between human fields. I have intellectualized the importance of this factor, yet I have been trying to *apply* my energy field topically, like a hot pack! Ah-ha!

Looking further, I realize that I have been involved in egocentric exercises instead of in dynamic activity. I recognize a fear of failure, but so what? In order to be a healer, one must risk violating the field boundaries of self and others. As a nurse, I have impinged upon the human field integrity of others with other "things": medications, instruments, treatments such as electroshock therapy and insulin shock therapy, and so on, but for some reason I have to rationalize conscious, direct, and open investment of my own self in the healing process. Self-investment connotes an unsurpassable commitment. Do I believe adequately in myself to develop the ability to make this self-projection with "effortless" effort?

J.R.A.

SOME EXPERIENCES IN THE USE OF THERAPEUTIC TOUCH

Rheumatoid Arthritis

One night, while on the 12 M–8 A.M. tour of duty, the call light went on in Room 9. I had expected it, and it was on schedule—every six hours. The patient, Mr. S., has Rheumatoid Arthritis. He is a young man in his early thirties and has a pleasant personality. In addition to the aspirin that he gets every four hours, he also gets another analgesic—Darvon, 100 mgm—every six hours if he needs it. I went to his room with the Darvon in my hand. He said that he was in pain and that his shoulders were very stiff. I suggested the idea of trying Therapeutic Touch first, and he was all for it. "I will try anything that can help me," he said. "I already have my own drug store here" (pointing to his abdomen).

When I started TT, I asked him to tell me any sensations he felt.

After a while he said, "I feel coolness in my left shoulder, and in my right shoulder I am getting a sensation I get every time I have a haircut." I asked him to gently move his shoulders, and he did so. Then he said, "My shoulders feel loose and the pain is gone. It must be psychological."

I, myself, was not sure whether Therapeutic Touch really worked on him. He might be trying to be nice to me by assuring me that I had done a successful treatment. I did not want him to be in pain for the rest of the night, so I left the medication by his bedside with the instruction that he take it any time he want to.

Three hours passed. Mr. S. was sound asleep, and the Darvon was still on the bedside table. In the morning, five hours after the treatment, Mr. S. was still asleep, but by this time the pill was gone.

Well, not bad for a start.

N.T.R.

Pain in An Ankle That Had Been Fractured

My girlfriend fractured her left ankle and wore a plaster cast for several weeks. After the cast was removed, she claimed that she was never free from pain. One day, she came to my apartment, and I saw her limping. I asked her if I could do Therapeutic Touch to her ankle, and she consented.

I held my hands about two to four inches from her. Over some areas of her leg, I felt a tremendous heat; and over one area I felt a sudden pulsation that caused my hands to bounce. I treated her for about fifteen minutes. She told me that she felt heat, a tingling sensation, and a feeling of relaxation. I advised her not to put any undue strain on the ankle.

On her way home, she forgot my warning, for she had to run about a half a block to catch her bus. While she was sitting comfortably on the bus, she suddenly realized that she was able to run and that her ankle was free of pain. She claimed that this was the first time her ankle had been painless since the fracture.

Muscle Spasm

I didn't have long to wait for my first opportunity to try Therapeutic Touch. My husband had a recurrence of muscle spasm in his back and was twisted with pain. I felt secure with him; I knew he would be accepting of what might seem strange to others. First I centered. . . . I was conscious of the space around us and of a tingling in the palms of my hands. I was not aware of the perceptions of the healee, only of the opportunity to help.

My husband seemed very relaxed—in fact, I was afraid that he had fallen asleep. He said he felt relaxed to the point of feeling "limp." Time had seemed to move very slowly, and I could not judge how long I worked, but I reached a point at which I stopped. There was no discernible reason; I just knew that it was over. It wasn't fatigue—it just stopped. My husband reported that he felt as though waves were flowing over him and through him and that, along with the deep relaxation, there was relief from the pain. He was able to stand straighter, and the previously spastic muscle was visibly relaxed.

Just a few weeks later, he pulled a hamstring muscle severely during a ball game. I was there, and, with Therapeutic Touch, he was able to stand and walk immediately, although with a limp, and he felt totally well in a day. Previously, when he had had the same type of injury, he was unable to do any weight-bearing activity for at least a day, and it usually took a week or more to heal.

E.S.

Pain of Neck, Shoulders and Cervical Spine

Ms. T. was suffering from pain of the neck, shoulders, and cervical spine and was willing to try TT. She found a comfortable position, and I placed my hands over the painful areas. I thought that by closing my eyes I would be able to pick up the cues better; and after a while, I began to feel a flow of heat along my arms to the palms of my hands, which I directed to the painful areas.

I asked her what she was feeling; and she said that at the beginning, she felt a prickling sensation that became a kind of heat radiation which produced a relaxing effect on her. At the same time, I had noticed that a sense of peace and relaxation had also pervaded my whole being.

I worked with this patient for four consecutive days for about fifteen minutes per day. Ms. T. was overwhelmed with the positive effect of the treatment. She felt considerable relief from the constant pain, and she claimed that now she could turn her head and bend without any pain at all.

V.G.C.

Stiffness and Soreness of the Shoulder

An orderly came to work last Monday with stiffness and soreness over his right shoulder. During the weekend, he had been playing tennis, and he was now in pain. I asked him if he would be willing to try TT. After my success with Ms. T. (see above), I had gained a lot of confidence in myself and wanted to help.

He was willing, and I applied Therapeutic Touch. To my astonishment, in no more than ten minutes, he verbalized the same experience that Ms. T. had had. He said that he felt an electric-like current penetrating his shoulder joint, and then the sensation of heat followed. This was accompanied by a sense of relaxation.

V.G.C.

Headache

On Saturday, a woman in my art class who knows that I am studying Therapeutic Touch told me that she had a headache, and she wanted me to make her feel better. Well, after centering myself, I did the whole routine, and the results were exciting. My friend said that she had felt a good deal of heat almost immediately. Then she said that she felt a pulling sensation through her head and out, and with it a feeling of relaxation at the back of her head, and then the pain was gone.

Not only did she feel better, but so did I!

B.B.

It was a terrible day, hectic and nervewracking, and one of my colleagues complained of headache. I said, "I'll take your headache away; I'll do Therapeutic Touch!" She laughed, was skeptical, and continued with her work. Two other friends, skeptics both, were there and they watched with amusement. Not getting an outright refusal, I decided to do what I could and put my hands over her neck, where the muscles seemed to be taut. You could tell from the way she sat, with her shoulders hunched up, that she was really up-tight. In retrospect, I should have scanned her field more thoroughly than the brief going over I gave it, but at any rate, before long she looked up from her work in wonderment and said, "I feel it! I feel the heat!" I continued for several more minutes, by which time she was truly astounded, for she now felt the heat radiating up and down her neck, and her headache was gone! It was just a great feeling for me—not only were they my friends, but they were also skeptics!

C.B.

Temperature Elevation in a Child

One night, my six-year-old daughter woke up crying. When I touched her forehead, I was horrified because it was so very hot. I became even more concerned when I took her temperature and saw the thermometer register 105°F. I immediately gave her a sponge bath and aspirin tablets. After fifteen minutes, I took her temperature again, but much to my disappointment it remained at 105°F.

I woke up my husband, and we took her to the emergency room of a nearby hospital. The physician on duty gave her elixir of phenobarbital to prevent convulsions and also gave her aspirin for the fever. He took off all her clothes and turned on the air conditioner in the room. We stayed for almost three hours, but the temperature of my daughter went down only one degree—to 104°F. We were finally told to go home and to see the child's private pediatrician.

It was not until we got home that I remembered your story about using the cotton on Joan, who had had a high temperature. I got out a piece of the cotton that I had previously energized and applied it and Therapeutic Touch to my daughter. Her temperature went down to 101°F; and after a half-hour, we took her to the pediatrician's office. She got a penicillin shot, oral antibiotic, and antipyretic medication, and we went home. As soon as we arrived home, I took her temperature again, and, to my relief, it was 99°F. I think that it was Therapeutic Touch that did the trick, for we live nearby the doctor's office, and there was very little time for the medication to work.

I.A.S.

Crying Babies

There were five pediatric patients who came to the operating room suite still crying, although they had all received preoperative sedatives one hour previously. To prove again if Therapeutic Touch would work, I did TT to see if we could eliminate the need for further medication. Three of these babies stopped crying and went to sleep; the other two seemed relaxed and did not cry any more.

V.G.C.

In my work as a clinical instructor, I continually move from patient to patient as I facilitate the acquiring of clinical skills, supervise patient care, and demonstrate technique. In a pediatric area, there are many infectious agents, and good handwashing technique is taught in the interest of reducing the possibility of cross-infection. Yet there are also these small human beings who can't understand their discomfort and who have no resources to draw upon to cope with the unfamiliarity of their environment. It is a deep and natural urge to comfort a crying infant or child, to establish contact, to support them in their anguish. But when more than one is crying, it can become a cruel delay to observe handwashing technique between contact with each child. It was out of this dilemma that a natural solution was employed—Therapeutic Touch.

The centering could be done quickly, and when it was accomplished, I gently modulated the energy flow from my hands. I "unruffled" the child's field without making body contact. I noticed that the child would become calm, stop crying, and then open his eyes wide for a moment, as if in recognition of some great truth sifting down through the collective unconscious of Man. The thought struck me that they seemed to be having a deep "ah-ha!" After this, they seemed to take a deep breath and fall asleep, and I'd move on to the next child.

E.S.

A Human Support System

The most moving experience I've ever had occurred two weeks ago while I was nursing a two-year-old critically ill baby boy. The baby was having an acute, severe, fatal reaction to a combination of chemotherapy and radiation therapy. He was actively bleeding from his lesions. He was irritable and restless and was having difficulty breathing. He was in fluid overload pending congestive heart failure and renal shutdown. I took one look at the child and left the room. I thought I would be sick. Oh, what medical monsters we can create!

I gathered my thoughts and went back determined to make this child as comfortable as possible. I spent the whole day talking with him, changing his bandages, doing as many comforting measures as I could think of. As I stood by his crib, he could sense my presence and would reach out for me. I wanted to transmit my calmness to him. His Mom helped me with his care, and he grew less irritable as he realized that his family was near. Emotions had a direct bearing on his energy. Bobby was more comfortable and more trusting; it was easier for him to breathe, and he slept deeply.

The second day, I listened to the report that death was imminent and that the family was crazy with grief. I again spent the morning with the family, reinforcing the fact that the situation was grave, but that I would not leave them alone.

By noon, Bobby was comfortable enough to sleep. Because he had not died during this critical time period, his chances for survival were improving. My intent was not to "save" Bobby from death; rather, it was to reduce the fear, panic, and tension in the environment that surrounded him. The way an individual perceives a threat is important to his dealing with it.

By late afternoon, one of the attending physicians commented to me about how much "better" Bobby had responded when I was there. I was trying so hard to be a human support system, to transfer potential energies within the human field. This is what nursing is all about to me. In attempting to transfer my strength to this baby, I was calling upon my experiences of perceptions, emotions, memories, and creative imagery, the tacit dimensions of my nursing interactions, and touch, which is the actualizer.

K.M.

My patient was a physician from South America who had malignant lymphoma. I felt particularly frustrated in caring for him because of a language barrier, for neither of us could understand the other and, in addition, there was that old bugaboo: "There is nothing more that can be done for him."

I decided that the least I could do was to clean his lesions and give him a backrub. As I went to get the materials, I thought of the principles of Therapeutic Touch that I could incorporate. I centered and proceeded to clean his lesions and then rub his back. I could feel "rough" areas in his field, and I "unruffled" them. He turned and looked at me, smiled, and closed his eyes with a sigh of serenity. During the Assessment and treatment, I could feel him relaxing.

I was the healer, but I was also relaxing; I was completely absorbed in what I was doing and felt at peace. My muscles were relaxed, I felt that my heart and respiratory rate were slower, and time itself seemed slower.

I had a visual image of my hands somehow "catching" and directing energy. Time, for me, was slower; I was involved in the moment, the "now." I ended the treatment, helped the patient put on a new gown, and wished him "Buenos noches." As I turned to leave, our eyes met, and he said, "Muchos gracias, senorita."

Every day on rounds, I went to his room, and he would point to his watch and then to his back, asking me what time I would be in. We had developed a rapport which transcended the spoken word. I also noticed that he stopped taking pain medication at bedtime. He never said that our sessions stopped the pain, in so many words; what I perceived was a deep relaxation response that helped him to sleep. I went away for a few days vacation, and when I returned, he had gone back to South America. I didn't save his life nor did I cure him, but I didn't fail.

C.H.

Stress

This was a specially interesting week for me, for I had a chance to practice Therapeutic Touch at work. One of the patients I had assigned to me had Down's Syndrome; she was mongoloid and about fifty-three years of age, and she had come to the hospital for eye surgery.

On the morning of the surgery, she was very frightened and would not let anyone near her. Six people had to hold her down so that the eye medication could be administered, after which she cried and screamed. In order to calm her, I had everyone leave the room, and I then placed my hands near her in Therapeutic Touch. I could feel much heat coming from her, which I "unruffled." After about ten minutes, she had stopped screaming and was quite relaxed and in charge of herself. My staff was impressed; the doctors were impressed; and I felt pretty good about it, too.

E.K.

I work as a surgical staff nurse in one of the big hospitals here in Manhattan. A male patient, Mr. F., was admitted to our unit with a diagnosis of left inguinal hernia. He was ninety-one years old, with a long history of alcoholism.

After undergoing several tests, the doctors found that he had a tumor in his bowel. His surgery was delayed because of the patient's nutritional status and the surgical risk involved. However, in a short while, Mr. F. developed an intestinal obstruction, and he had to be operated on. One of the results of that surgery was a colostomy. Postoperatively, he had circulatory problems and developed a pneumonia, so that he had to stay in the surgical intensive care unit for three weeks. Prior to surgery, Mr. F. was alert and coherent and was quite an independent man. When he came back to our floor, he was confused and disoriented, continuously saying, "May I help?" almost twenty-four hours a day. He sounded like a broken record.

When I first saw Mr. F., I knew then that I would like him; I felt close to him—for no reason I know. Other patients complained of Mr. F.'s constant noise. The staff tried to orient him to his environment, but to no avail. The doctors bypassed his room during rounds because they couldn't get any logical information from him. I pitied Mr. F. and wanted to help him.

After I finished giving Mr. F. a bath on the day he was assigned to me, I decided to try Therapeutic Touch. Most of the interaction was concerned with "unruffling" the field and helping it to return to balance.

The next day, it was reported that Mr. F. had been quiet the entire night. We made rounds, and, to our surprise, Mr. F. was sitting at the side of his bed, his feet dangling. He smiled at us when we entered the room and said, "Good morning."

My coworkers commented that Mr. F. had decided to wake up, but I was puzzled. Was the intervention with Therapeutic Touch of significance here? There had been no change in the medical regime, and I decided to continue TT.

His progress was such that the doctors decided to transfer Mr. F. to a nursing home. Unfortunately, he developed a pneumonia, and consequent urinary tract complications followed very quickly. He became weak and pale and refused to eat. Previously, he would accept TT gladly, but now he refused with a grim determination.

One day, I was trying to feed him when he suddenly became very pale, his breathing was labored, and he was barely responsive. We put him back to bed; this time, he had no energy to resist TT. After the treatment, his breathing returned to normal, he regained his color, and he fell asleep.

I was off the following day, and when I reported back to work, the night nurse told me that Mr. F. had died early that morning. It did not make me feel bad. Deep inside, I felt that I had helped him. In spite of the infections he had, he did not have a fever, he was not in agony, and he died peacefully.

A.B.

My next positive experience with Therapeutic Touch was in relation to Mr. S., a sixty-five-year-old man in the terminal stages of cancer. He would moan constantly, with or without medication. His wife sat by his side all day. She was in an extreme state of anxiety and would come running for help every time he moved, made a different sound, or changed his breathing pattern.

I decided to try to help Mr. S. by doing TT while I was washing him that morning. Ms. S. was in the room, hovering nervously. I held my hands over his spine, where the pain seemed most intense, and I could feel an energy flow from my palms. Almost immediately, he stopped moaning and became very relaxed and peaceful. I also felt a sense of closeness, a unity with him, a calm sense of peacefulness. His wife, sitting in a chair nearby, also became very relaxed. The external environment seemed to all flow together, boundaries meshed, time seemed to stand still. The imagery in my head was of unity, of oneness, of a flowing, rhythmic togetherness. I could tell when the healing act was completed: The unity began to separate, boundaries materialized, and the spell was broken, so to speak. After this treatment, Mr. S. slept quietly without moaning. His wife became very calm and relaxed, sitting quietly by his side, with her hand in his. It seemed very peaceful.

Mr. S. died two days later, his wife at his bedside. She had remained very calm during the two days. Now she was crying softly, but she seemed resigned. I felt as though I had treated her, too.

J.M.

The most recent patient I worked with was a man considered by his physicians to be terminal. Among his problems were severe electrolyte imbalance, and therefore he was frequently confused and restless. As I dislike to use restraints and rarely give sedatives unless I've exhausted other possibilities, I decided to use Therapeutic Touch to help him. His entire field was so disturbed that it took longer than usual to "unruffle" it, but once I did I could feel him begin to relax. However, he never did relax completely, although I tried and tried.

After two treatments, when he still didn't fully relax, I found that I was beginning to get angry. I had helped before, why not now? With thoughts like this running around in my head, I suddenly stopped short. Who did I think I was? Therapeutic Touch wasn't something that you turned on, like a light, that was guaranteed to work every time. Was I thinking more about the satisfaction I got out of the treatment than about the patient? With this thought in mind, I was able to resume the treatment, but now, after having confronted myself, it was with a sense of peace.

Combining TT with the sparing use of sedatives, which only seemed to add to his confusion, helped the patient to remain calm and collected, and so we never did have to use the restraints. He died a peaceful, dignified death last Sunday.

C.H.

Self Healing

Initially, I decided to perform Therapeutic Touch on myself when I experienced severe, cramping abdominal pain, which was unrelieved in spite of my having taken Darvon and two aspirin tablets. As my discomfort increased, and with no one whom I could call on for help, I decided to lie on my couch, relax, and center, and then I did Therapeutic Touch to myself. As I lightly passed my hands over my abdomen, where I had been feeling unmitigated pain, I experienced a sense of intense heat in my right palm. I am unsure if the heat radiated from my abdomen or from my hand; however, after engaging in TT for two to three minutes, I found that the pain had dissipated, much to my astonishment.

E.G.

I am convinced that every accident-prone person needs to include Therapeutic Touch in his repertoire. To wit:

On Monday, I smashed my left index finger with the kitchen closet door, and the pain was excruciating. Ah-ha! thought I, Therapeutic Touch is what I need at a time like this. After two to three minutes of TT on my finger, the pain was completely relieved.

On Wednesday morning, as I was getting out of the shower, I brushed my left upper arm across the hot water pipe. I didn't actually burn my arm, but it was quite painful to touch. Once again, TT came to the rescue: Almost instantly, my pain was relieved.

On Thursday, my husband and I were crossing a street in Chinatown, and I tripped and twisted my left ankle and fell to the ground. By the time we reached the car, my ankle was really throbbing, and it looked as though we would have to postpone dinner. However, once again Therapeutic Touch came to the rescue, and we went off to dinner in style.

Do you think we can bottle this and sell it to insurance companies?

N.O.N.

Inanimate Objects

The term "human field" has been used many times on these pages without specific definition. I don't think we have an adequate definition, for there are too many unknowns about the human condition at this time. As stated earlier, I conceptualize the human field as a nexus of many fields of which Man is the test object, so to speak, analogous to the concept of the particle of matter in quantum theory that is thought to be but a momentary manifestation, a result of interacting fields.[11] Within this context, it seems to me that Man is able to interact with many fields—many more than any living creature—and that may be why he has been in the forefront of evolution here on Earth. It is, therefore, not surprising to me that we can interact with inanimate objects as a field phenomenon—that is, at a distance, as in psychokinesis where a person can influence objects from afar. It is, after all, not unusual to kick a car tire in desperation on a frigid or rainy morning and find that a previously balky motor engine turns over, sometimes with the most modest of apologetic coughs.

Something like this happened to me one time; you might find it amusing. I went to visit a group of physicists in San Francisco who were doing various parapsychological investigations. They showed me around their workshops, and I was very impressed by a large, walk-in Faraday cage which had, as I understood it, been set up to eliminate interaction with the electromagnetic field. I noticed a small black boxlike affair on a

[11] Victor Giullemin, *The Story of Quantum Mechanics* (New York: Charles Scribner's Sons, 1968), p. 175.

table inside the cage which had what seemed to be a circular antenna, perhaps five to six inches in diameter, coming from it. Outside the cage was a series of shiny new electronic instrumentations with many attachments. I asked what was the purpose of the cage and machinery. "Why don't you step inside and find out for yourself?" said Henry, my host.

I stepped into the cage. Immediately, the consoles came alive with high-pitched electronic beeps, and I could see the green light from a viewing screen of some kind go on. I walked towards the table and sat down, and immediately the beeps stopped. "Ah-ha!" thought I, "The beeps must have to do with movement." After sitting there quietly for a moment, wondering what the black boxlike affair on the table in front of me was, I decided to see how it would react to Therapeutic Touch. I placed my hands on either side of the black box and, without moving them further, I proceeded to set up a localized field between the two *chakras* in the palms of my hands. Immediately, the electronic monster gave voice to the incessant beeps. I have studied the effects of mantras, which are specifically voiced sounds, for many years, and I decided to see what effect the mantra *Aum* might have on the situation. I therefore continued the field while I sounded the *Aum*. The beeping stopped. Henry turned, left the room, and returned with three other physicists. "Can you do that again?" he asked. "I can try," I answered, and I repeated the performance. The fellows all seemed to start to talk at once. Apparently, they were interested in what they were saying—all Greek to me—for they went off to another workroom still loudly discussing—whatever. When I got out of the cage and went upstairs, I found myself caught up in elaborate plans to have lunch at a storefront deli, and I never did find out what their opinion of the whole affair was.

Pat, one of the Krieger's Krazies, had a different experience. She worked in the labor and delivery room of a large hospital in New York City. On her rounds one day, she found that another Krieger's Krazy, Carol, was in the labor room expecting her baby.

As she came into the room, she noticed that the fetal monitor, a machine that electronically reflects the condition of the unborn child, was very noisy. She and Carol discussed the noisy machine, and Pat tried to fix it, but to no avail. Conversation turned to Carol's condition. Carol was experiencing considerable pressure and asked Pat to do Therapeutic Touch on her. Pat, who had just recently started to learn TT, panicked and said, "I'm just beginning. I'm not sure," and she hurriedly left the room.

Once in the nursing office, she realized her fear and the confusion it had caused her. She went back to Carol's room, apologized, and said that she'd be glad to do TT if Carol told her what to do to relieve the pressure. She then put her hands a few inches from Carol's abdomen, and something happened that startled them both: Within moments, the noisy fetal monitor, which had previously been all but bouncing up and down with the vibrations of the noise, quieted down and acted quite normally from then on. Carol had a normal, natural delivery—a vibrant, bouncing baby, of course!

Conclusions, Comments, and Queries

The above incident could be a "cute" story, but there is more to tell. Pat's understanding of and ability to do Therapeutic Touch rapidly increased during the next several weeks. She became valued not only as a good nurse but for her increasing sensitivity to her patients' needs. These special qualities attracted the attention of one of the major gynecologists at the hospital at which she worked, and he chose her to participate with him in a special kind of delivery which was only the fifth of its kind in the past twenty years. This team effort has continued, and it is but one of several such happenings between health colleagues which combine both traditional and alternative modes of healing. This kind of team effort is useful, for a fractured bone will heal much more rapidly if it is set before TT is done, necrotic tissue will heal more rapidly, if deep seated pathology is resected first, and so on.

There are now many such Therapeutic Touch teams in hospitals around the country—Boston, New York City, Austin, Tucson, San Francisco, and Portland, Oregon, to name but a few. In some hospitals, Therapeutic Touch is used for its relaxation effect before the administration of anesthesia. It is also used in cardiac units previous to the insertion of cardiac pacemakers, and it is used on apprehensive patients who are to have dental procedures. The ability of TT (which is frequently written as π, the Greek letter *pi* in order books) to alleviate pain is used to advantage in emergency rooms while waiting for a medical prescription to be written; as a matter of fact, its use as such has given rise to an "in" expression for TT. It is called: "What to do until the doctor comes." Its enhancement of wound healing is widely known and is implemented in many settings. As noted previously, the safety level of Therapeutic

Touch for both healer and healee has been excellent, and this accounts for much of its enthusiastic acceptance. It is an holistic act, and its practice can be a significant growth experience.

Although most of the anecdotes in this book concern professional persons in the health field, the points of entry to Therapeutic Touch occur at all levels. Wherever you are, you can help.

There are still many unknowns about the dyadic interaction between healer and healee, and intelligent caution is a wise stance. For myself, I still pursue the question, "Why is touch therapeutic?" in continued research. However, no amount of intellectualization will do the trick; the ultimate nature of Therapeutic Touch is experiential; and so my final words to you are: *practice, practice, practice.* You can help, and you can heal—but only if you understand what it is you are doing.

Appendix 1:

Experiential Criteria during Therapeutic Touch

Directions: Please fill out the following questions as fully as you are able. Use additional paper as necessary.

During the healing act of Therapeutic Touch:

1. *How do you sense the external environment—that is, is there any significant difference in the manner in which you perceive things and/or people around you?*

____

____

____

____

2. Do you feel any significant changes in your heart rate or respiratory rate or in your body muscle tone or sense of energy flow?

____

____

____

____

3. In what way would you describe how you get meaning from your experience—that is, are you able to recapture the internal dialogue that goes on inside of you when you try to explain to yourself what it is your senses are telling you?

____

____

____

____

4. Have you noticed any significant changes in your emotions?

____

____

____

____

5. In what way do you use your memory—for instance, are you aware of a continuity of experience?

6. Does any change occur in your sense of time; for example, does time speed up or slow down?

7. What sense of identity have you—that is, what role do you perceive yourself enacting?

8. Are there significant changes in your evaluative and cognitive processes—that is, do you think in a different way during Therapeutic Touch?

9. How do you perceive your body image—that is, what feedback do you get from the movements, postures, and energetic flow from your body?

Appendix II:

The Two Endpoints of an EEG Continuum of Meditation—Alpha/Theta and Fast Beta

ABSTRACT

In this case study, the psychophysiological changes associated with a type of meditation called Therapeutic Touch were examined. One Therapeutic Touch healer was studied for two days, alone, and with three patients. EEG, GSR, EKG and temperature were recorded. The main finding was a preponderance of fast beta EEG activity present in the healer. The physiological results are interpreted as representative of this type of meditative

Reprinted with permission of the authors: Sonia Ancoli, Langely Porter Neuropsychiatric Institute, University of California, San Francisco. Eric Peper, Ph. D., Center for Interdisciplinary Sciences, San Francisco State University, San Francisco.

process. Problems involved in this type of research and suggestions for future research are discussed.

The physiological parameters recorded during meditative practices usually follow the direction of low arousal patterns. For example, the EEG during meditation often shows an increase in alpha and an enhancement of theta electroencephalographic (EEG) activity (Kasamatsu & Hirai, 1969). Yet alpha and theta EEG activity are only part of the many different physiological responses observed during meditation. Das and Gastaut (1955), Peper and Pollini (1976), and Banquet (1973) have observed an enhancement of synchronous beta EEG patterns in advanced meditators. We hypothesize that the different physiological observations are probably related to the *style* of the specific meditative process; with alpha theta EEG low arousal as one endpoint of a continuum and fast frequency beta EEG at the other.

The purposes of this paper are to:

1. Present a hypothesis that EEG findings in meditation are on a continuum. One locus is alpha/theta activity as reported in a number of meditation studies (Chhina & Singh, 1961; Banquet, 1973; Kasamatsu & Hirai, 1969; Wallace and Benson, 1972); the other is a fast frequency beta, previously cited by Das & Gastaut (1955), reobserved by Peper and Pollini (1976), and reobserved in this case study.
2. Report the observation that fast EEG activity is associated with Therapeutic Touch (fast EEG activity can also be defined as beta or synchronous beta EEG activity with a frequency range of 18–20 Hz).
3. Speculate on the meaning of beta EEG frequency as compared to the usual findings of alpha and theta EEG activity in meditation, and on how this may relate to the meditative process.
4. Suggest ways by which the psychophysiological outcome can be used to authenticate the meditative process and to use it as a tool to assist learning of the meditative process.
5. Examine the psychophysiological changes that occurred during the healing meditation (Therapeutic Touch).
6. Suggest new strategies by which meditators can be studied.

This research note reports data from a single advanced meditator,

Dr. Dolores Krieger (DK), who practices a meditation known as "Therapeutic Touch" (Krieger, 1976). Therapeutic Touch has within it components of "the laying-on of hands" and "bedside manner." DK teaches this healing meditation at the New York University Division of Nursing, and she has practiced it for many years.

DK described that, in the process of Therapeutic Touch, the healer becomes quiet, passively listens with her hands, and gently attunes herself to the patient. The healer places her hands upon the areas of "accumulated tension" in the patient and redirects these energies. In the process of touching, the healer reports that she uses herself as a model to "input energy" to help the healee rise to a level of comparative energy.

This is a complex form of meditative practice which involves the control of body energy centers known as *chakras* (Govinda, 1976; Govinda, 1969; Evans-Wentz, 1967).

With Therapeutic Touch, as with other meditative practices, one focuses without effort: The mind is totally focused upon the healing touch, and no other thoughts enter awareness. Meditation is mindfulness ("attentiveness training"), a process not usually taught in our educational system. As the following exercise illustrates, when we do a task, extraneous thoughts usually enter unaware and we are not mindful:

> Sit quietly and, for the next two minutes, look at your thumbnail. Observe it lovingly, do not judge it. Behold the thumbnail in active contemplation. At the end of two minutes, recount how many critical or unaware extraneous thoughts occurred.

With sustained practice, mindfulness can be achieved, and the number of distracting thoughts will be reduced, while the meditator's mind stays alert and passively focused.

PROBLEMS IN THIS TYPE OF RESEARCH

There are major problems in studying adept meditators, especially single subjects. (Some comparable problems in biofeedback have been described elsewhere (Peper, 1976a, 1976b)).

1. The process is idiosyncratic, and it may not be possible to generalize it or to replicate it with other individuals.

2. The conditions of baseline, experimental sessions, and post-baseline are artificial boundaries which the experimenter sets up. For the adept subject, these dichotomies and distinctions may not exist. For example, DK uses the Therapeutic Touch process as soon as she is seated quietly with the patient; Therapeutic Touch *implies* becoming aware of the patient. This process is automatic for her. She starts attuning to the patient the moment he/she enters. Hence, a "baseline condition" is actually a combined process of that baseline *plus* the healing meditation.
3. There may be no change in physiological functioning in a subject who for years has attuned herself to be in a different state of awareness. For her, there is no longer a difference between meditative and nonmeditative states.

Only a longitudinal study would indicate the physiological transformations of a meditator, a study which to date has not been done. However, a comparative study demonstrating EEG differences of alpha EEG amplitude and theta EEG trains has been reported with beginning and adept Zen meditators and with nonmeditators (Kasamatsu & Hirai, 1969).

PATIENTS

Three patients were monitored while DK practiced Therapeutic Touch. They were: HP, a sixty-year-old male with a five-year history of severe neck, back, and head pain; JB, a thirty-year-old female with a history of fibroid cysts in her breasts; and RG, a twenty-three-year-old female with a three-year history of severe chronic migraine as well as one grand mal seizure. A fourth subject, AB, with a history of severe backache, was eliminated, because she was afraid that participation would jeopardize her workmen's compensation claim.

METHODS

DK was studied for two consecutive days. On Day 1, baseline levels were recorded from DK alone. Since most of the healing was done while DK was standing, data was collected for eyes open and closed, while sitting and standing.

Different electrode configurations were used to explore the Therapeutic Touch process. Grass cup electrodes and Grass electrode paste were used for bipolar EEG configurations located at O_2, O_1, F_{p_1}, and F_{p_2}, and the mid-points between (P_4–C_4), (C_4–F_4), (P_3–C_3), and (C_3–F_3) with the earlobe as ground (Jasper, 1958). The electrooculograms (EOG) were recorded with slow or nonpolarizing biopotential skin electrodes (Beckman) attached to the outer and inner canthi of each eye. In addition, frontalis electromyographic (EMG) and left palmar galvanic skin response (GSR) leads were recorded. The EEG (O_1–P_3 and O_2–P_4) wrist to wrist heart rate (EKG), palmar GSR and temperature from the hands were also monitored for each patient.

APPARATUS

All recordings were done with the subjects in a softly-lit, electrically shielded, sound-deadened acoustical chamber. The patients were either sitting or in the prone position, with DK alternating between sitting and standing. All recordings were done on a Grass model 78D polygraph with four model 7P511G amplifiers, two wide-band AC pre-amplifier integrators (model 7P3B), and two low-level DC pre-amplifiers (model 7P1E). Sixty-Hz filters were used for each channel. (However, this did not filter out fast EEG frequencies.) In addition, the data from Day 1 was recorded on a Vetter Model A tape recorder.

RESULTS

The major observation was DK's EEG record. Regardless of the experimental condition, it showed a preponderance of fast synchronous EEG activity, often embedded in a mixed EEG record, as is illustrated in Figure 1.[1] Since fast rhythmic EEG activity would be confused with

[1] Even though fast beta EEG activity is often associated with certain medications (such as barbiturates) (Kooi, 1971), DK was not taking any medication.

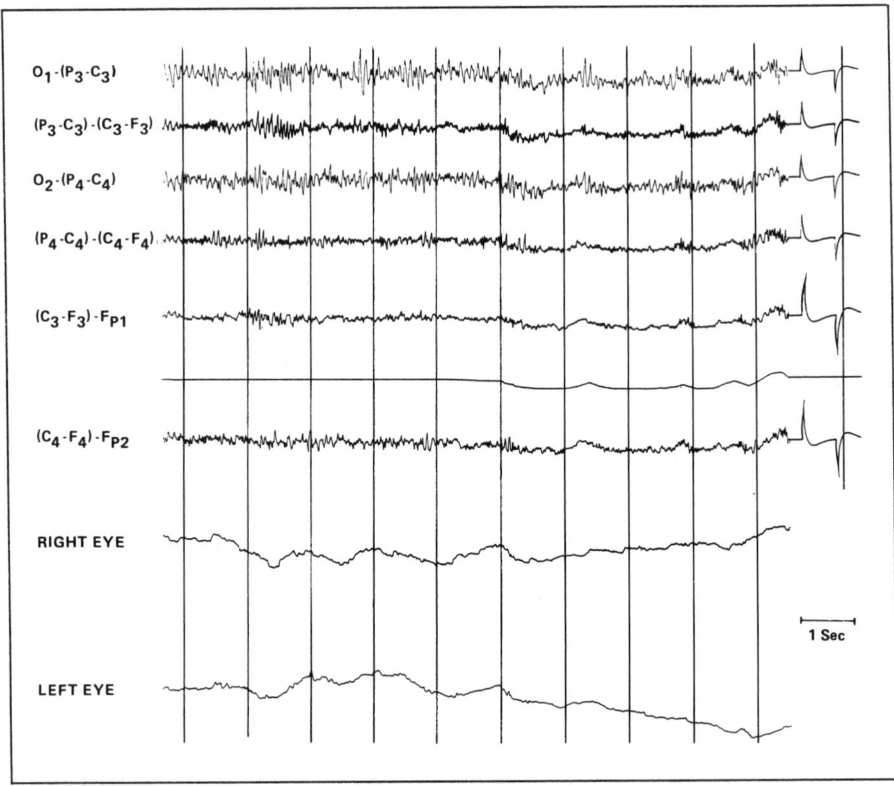

Figure A-1. EEG and EOG recording of DK during eyes-open, baseline. Note the preponderance of fast EEG (50 uV calibration).

EMG activity, DK's frontalis EMG was compared with her EEG. As seen in Figure 2, fast EEG activity was also present during low frontalis EMG.

The EEG recording indicated that DK was not actively attending to outside cues. The EOG recording showed that her eyes were slightly diverged and showed *no* movement (i.e., no slow rolling or saccadic movements) during Therapeutic Touch unless she shifted positions (see Figure 3).

No major changes were seen in the patients' EEG, EKG, EMG, temperature, or GSR. All three patients basically showed a relaxed state with an abundance of large amplitude alpha activity, both with eyes open and eyes closed (see Figure 2). This was present in the baseline and did not change during the assessment or healing. All three patients reported that the Therapeutic Touch was relaxing and that they would again volunteer.

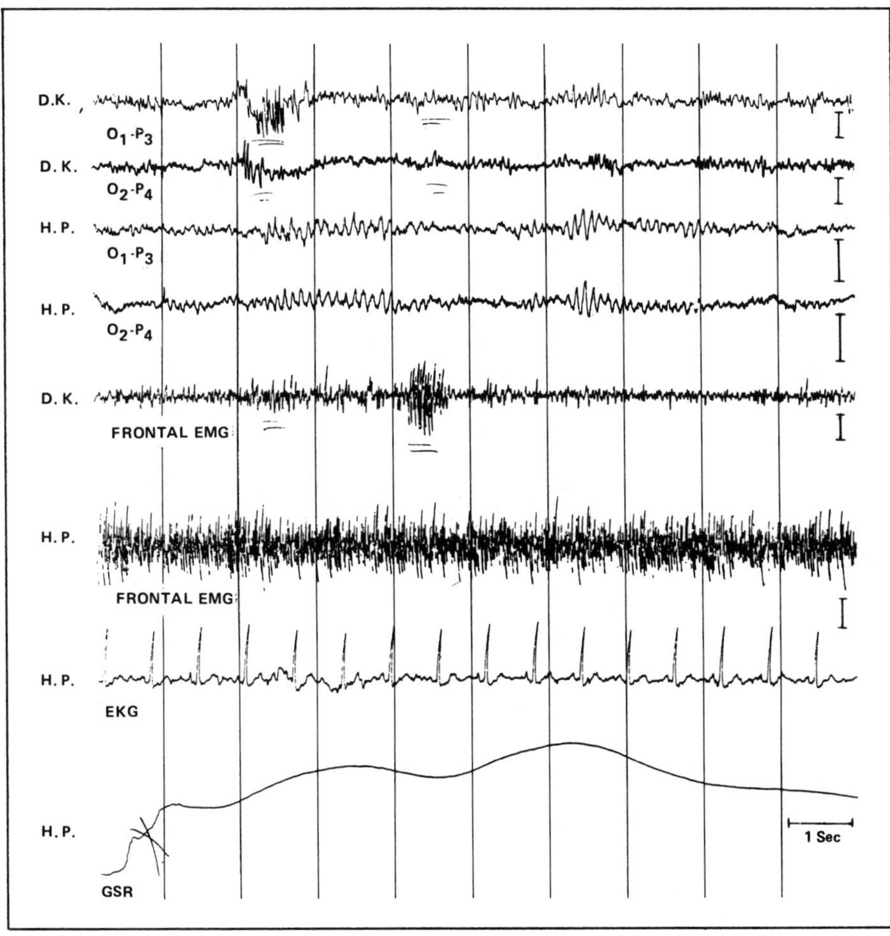

Figure A-2. EEG and EMG recording during the therapeutic touch. Simultaneous recording of the patient (HP) and healer (DK). Observe that increase in DK's fast beta EEG is not *associated with an increase in EMG. Also note the preponderance of alpha in the EEG of HP (50 uV calibration).*

We do not know to what extent the improvement of the patients was related to the Therapeutic Touch experience, because the study was *not* intended to test whether Therapeutic Touch had healing effect. In order to study the healing properties of Therapeutic Touch, controlled studies need to be done. The patients who participated in this study were nominally screened for existing pathology.

The improvement may not be related to the Therapeutic Touch experience, and no claims can be made. However, the experience was important to the patients. As RG pointed out, "This was the first time

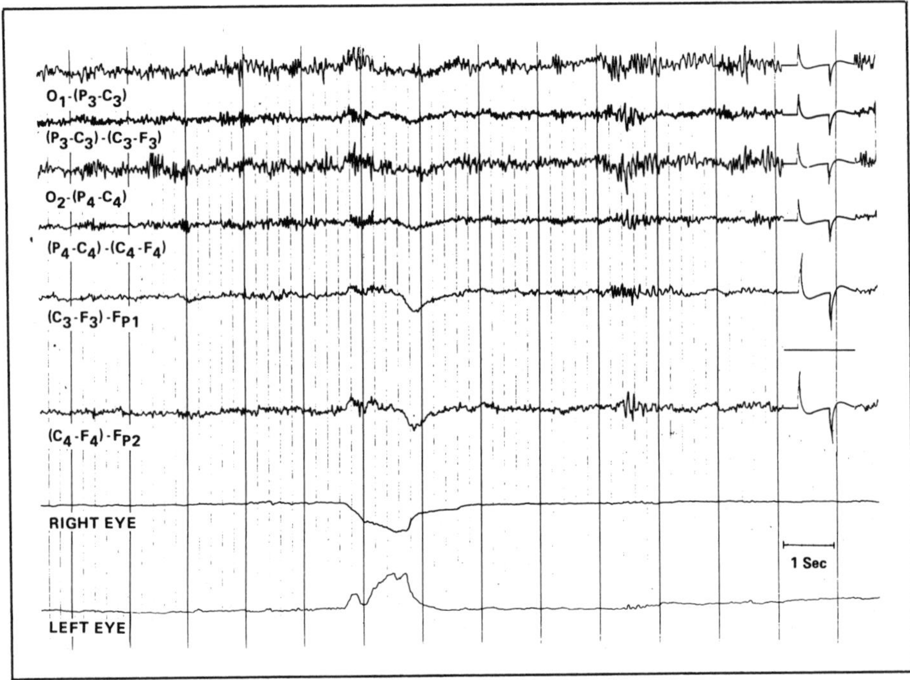

Figure A–3. EEG and EOG recording of DK during therapeutic touch. Note the preponderance of fast beta EEG and the extremely stable eye position. Eye movement occurred only when DK moved or shifted position (50 uV calibration).

that I felt that somebody (DK) really cared. It is so rare that somebody cares in a medical setting. In addition, I had tried to do something for myself. This made me feel better." Possibly, Therapeutic Touch could be a technique to investigate placebo dynamics.

DISCUSSION

The fast synchronous EEG activity recorded from DK is *striking* and *contrary* to the commonly accepted finding that the EEG of meditators is associated with an increase of alpha and theta activity. There are a number of possibilities as to why fast EEG is not usually associated with meditation.

1. It is present in other meditators but not usually observed.
2. It is a parameter of an unstudied meditation process.
3. It is idiosyncratic to DK.

The fast beta EEG activity may be more common than previously reported. Past research often could not observe this phenomenon because EEG was not analyzed for fast frequencies. In most studies of meditation, low pass filters were used, which filtered out frequencies greater than 15 Hz, therefore masking the observation of fast beta frequencies (Peper & Pollini, 1976). In addition, the data from EEG feedback studies are also meaningless, since in most studies alpha was defined, but beta and theta were seen as "not alpha" (Peper, 1974; Ancoli & Kamiya, 1977).

The fast beta activity is probably not idiosyncratic to DK, since fast beta activity and a decrease in alpha EEG activity have been reported in other meditators and most likely are associated with their particular meditative style (Das & Gastaut, 1955; Banquet, 1973; Peper & Pollini, 1976).

The predominant presence of beta in DK's EEG during her meditation may represent the physiological style of her meditation. For example, in meditation such as raja yoga, one can meditate upon a word or mantra. However, as one meditates upon the mantra, the "mind" may get distracted. One can be distracted by an itch or by hypnogogic imagery. This drifting may account for the high percentage of alpha and theta as well as for the Stage 1 sleep spindles observed in transcendental meditation (TM) meditators (Pagano, Rose, Stivers & Warrenburg, 1975). However, meditation can also be focused passive attention, in which the mind is so well trained that the moment one sits quietly and meditates, *no* extraneous images or thoughts come in; one is totally attentive without effort.

For DK, extraneous thoughts are no problem. She focuses without effort. As she reports, there are no longer ever any extraneous thoughts when she meditates—she passed through that process many years ago. Her eyes would focus at nothing in the distance so that she could passively attend to the sensation of the Therapeutic Touch experience (Figure 3). This carried over into her baseline periods. We interpret the presence of fast EEG activity in the subject as a learned passive control over her meditation to such an extent that she is totally focused and alert without ever drifting into hypnogogic imagery. We suspect that it is not the type of meditation that a person does that is important but rather *how* the person does it. For example, the person's mind (internal dialogue) is totally quiet. There are no extraneous thoughts while the person is focusing *passively with intention* upon a task.

When past psychophysiological data were recorded during meditation, the concurrent subjective reports or experiences were often lacking. This made any subjective interpretation of the data impossible. We suggest that fast EEG activity may be used in combination with subjective reports to identify the style of an advanced meditator. The study of meditation must account for these psychophysiological (EEG) differences. This can be done by grouping meditators into those who show a preponderance of fast beta EEG activity during meditation and those who show an increase in slow alpha/theta EEG activity. This type of research would help to clarify the hypothesis that fast beta EEG indicates a passive-focused attention without interruptive thoughts, a meditative state separate from the usual alpha/theta EEG state in which some subjects allow themselves to drift into quiet pleasantness.

We hope that this report will suggest and encourage a more precise investigation of meditation, both by studying the quality of the meditative experience and concurrently initiating an open-ended psychophysiological recording in order to avoid some of the pitfalls we have encountered.

We suggest that future research in Therapeutic Touch and meditation:

1. Look for other healers and meditators and for similar psychophysiological patterns.
2. Explore new baseline paradigms so that the meditation is not confounded with the baseline condition, such as by having the patient and the healer in separate rooms, or by giving the meditator an active task to keep him from meditating.
3. Look at additional physiological measures for the relaxation response in the patient.
4. Feedback those components of the physiological response that were most meaningful to the meditative experience of the subjects. Both patients and healers could describe which feedback signal was associated with the healing qualities of the meditation.
5. Initiate EEG feedback training with subjects in order to explore the subjective and objective experience of fast EEG beta activity.
6. Include spectral analysis of the EEG data in order to explore and understand the exact frequency distribution more fully.

SUMMARY

A pilot investigation of Therapeutic Touch indicated that the healer showed a preponderance of fast EEG activity. This data suggests that EEG changes may be linked to attentive meditation styles.

REFERENCES

ANCOLI, S., and KAMIYA, J. 1977. Methodological issues in alpha biofeedback training. *Proceedings of the Biofeedback Society of America.*

BANQUET, J.P. 1973. Spectral analysis of the EEG in meditation. *Electroenceph. Clin. Neurophysiol.*35:143–151.

DAS, N.N., and GASTAUT, H. 1955. Variations de l'activite electrique du cerveau, du couer et des muscles sequielettiques au cours de la meditation et de "l'extase" yoguique. *Electroenceph. Clin. Neurophysiol.* Supplement 6:211–219.

EVANS-WENTZ, W.Y., ed. 1967. *Tibetan yoga and secret doctrines* (2d ed.). London: Oxford University Press.

GOVINDA, LAMA A. 1969. *Foundations of Tibetan mysticism.* London: Rider & Co.

——. 1976. *Creative meditation and multidimensional consciousness.* Wheaton: Theosophical Publishing House.

JASPER, H.H. 1958. Report of the committee on methods of clinical examination in electroencephalography. *Electroenceph. Clin. Neurophysiol.* 10:371–375.

KASAMATSU, A., and HIRAI, T. 1969. An electroencephalographic study of the Zen meditation (Zazen). In C.G. Tart, ed. *Altered states of consciousness.* New York: Wiley.

KOOI, K.A. 1971. *Fundamentals of electroencephalography.* New York: Harper.

KRIEGER, D. 1976. Healing by the laying-on of hands as a facilitator of bioenergetic exchange: The response of in-vivo human hemoglobin. *International Journal for Psychoenergetic Systems.* 2:

PAGANO, R.R., ROSE, R.M., STIVERS, R.M., and WARRENBURG, W.S. 1975. Sleep during transcendental meditation. *Science* 191: 308.

PEPER, E. 1974. Problems in heart rate and alpha electroencephalographic feedback: Is the control over the feedback stimulus meaningful? *Kybernetik* 14:217-221.

——. 1976a. Problems in biofeedback training: An experiential analogy—urination. *Perspectives in Biology and Medicine* 19:402-412.

——. 1976b. Passive attention: The gateway to consciousness and autonomic control. In P.G. Zimbardo and F.L. Ruch, eds. *Psychology and life*. Chicago: Scott Foresman.

PEPER, E., and POLLINI, S.J. 1976. Fast beta activity: Recording limitations, problems and subjective reports. In *Proceedings of the Biofeedback Research Society*, Colorado Springs.

WALLACE, R.K. and H. BENSON. 1972. The physiology of meditation. *Scientific American* (February), pp. 84-90.

We appreciate the cooperation and discussion with Drs. Joe Kamiya, and Dolores Krieger, Joanne Kamiya, Jim Johnston, and the helpful assistance of Christopher Brown, Noel Mapstead, Tamar Morgan, Dr. Karen Naifeh, and Laura Stratachik. Reprint requests may be addressed to Erik Peper, Ph.D., 2236 Derby Street, Berkeley, CA 94705.